The Comfort of Home™
for Parkinson Disease

A Guide for Caregivers

The Comfort of Home caregiver book series is written for family and paraprofessional home caregivers who face the responsibilities of caring for aging friends, family, or clients. The disease-specific editions, often in collaboration with organizations supporting those conditions, address caregivers assisting people with those diseases.

Other Caregiver Resources from CareTrust Publications:

The Comfort of Home™: *A Complete Guide for Caregivers—Third Edition*
La comodidad del hogar™ *(Spanish Edition)*
The Comfort of Home™ *Multiple Sclerosis Edition*
The Comfort of Home™ *for Stroke: A Guide for Caregivers*
The Comfort of Home™ *for Chronic Lung Disease: A Guide for Caregivers*
The Comfort of Home™ *for Alzheimer's Disease: A Guide for Caregivers*
The Comfort of Home™ *Caregiving Journal*
The Comfort of Home™ *Caregivers—Let's Take Care of You!* Meditation CD

Newsletters:

The Comfort of Home™ *Caregiver Assistance News*
The Comfort of Home™ *Grand-Parenting News*
The Comfort of Home™ *Caregivers—Let's Take Care of You!*

Visit www.comfortofhome.com for forthcoming editions and other caregiver resources.

The Comfort of Home™

of Home™ for Parkinson Disease

A Guide for Caregivers

Maria M. Meyer

and

Paula Derr, RN, BSN, CEN, CCRN

with

Susan C. Imke, RN, MS

CareTrust Publications LLC
"Caring for you...caring for others."
Portland, Oregon

The Comfort of Home™ for Parkinson Disease: A Guide for Caregivers

Published by: CareTrust Publications LLC
P.O. Box 10283
Portland, Oregon 97296-0283
(800) 565-1533
Fax (503) 221-7019

Publisher's Cataloging-in-Publication
(Provided by Quality Books, Inc.)

Meyer, Maria M., 1948-
    The comfort of home for Parkinson disease : a guide
for caregivers / Maria M. Meyer and Paula Derr ; with
Susan C. Imke.
    p. cm.
    Includes index.
    ISBN 0-9664767-7-8

    1. Home care services—Handbooks, manuals, etc.
2. Caregivers—Handbooks, manuals, etc. 3. Parkinson's
disease.   I. Derr, Paula.   II. Imke, Susan C.
III. Title.

RA645.3.M496 2007   649.8
                       QBI06-600541

Cover Art and Text Illustration: Stacey L. Tandberg
Interior Design: Frank Loose
Cover Design: David Kessler
Page Layout: International Graphic Services

Distributed to the Trade by Publishers Group West.
Printed in the United States of America.

07 08 09 10 11 / 10 9 8 7 6 5 4 3 2 1

About the Authors

Maria Meyer has been a long-time advocate of social causes, beginning with her work as cofounder of the Society for Abused Children of the Children's Home Society of Florida. She was also founding executive director of the Children's Foundation of Greater Miami. Maria continued her work in institutional advancement for nonprofit organizations, ranging from homeless shelters to botanic gardens. When her father-in-law suffered a stroke in 1993, Maria became aware of the need for more information about how to care for an aging parent. That led Maria to found CareTrust Publications LLC, a company dedicated to producing reader-friendly books that help ordinary people cope with their increasing responsibilities for family members and friends. She and her husband also founded CareTrust Services LLC, an advisory firm that helps faith-based organizations develop affordable housing and assisted living for the elderly. Maria is the Northern California State Coordinator for the National Family Caregivers Association. She is a keynote speaker and workshop leader on caregiver topics to health care professionals and community groups, as well as a Caregiver Community Action Network volunteer for the National Family Caregiver Association.

Paula Derr has been employed by the Sisters of Providence Health System for over 25 years and is clinical educator for three emergency departments in the Portland metropolitan area. She is co-owner of InforMed, which publishes emergency medical services field guides for emergency medical technicians (EMTs), paramedics, firefighters, physicians, and nurses and has co-authored numerous health care articles. For Paula, home care is a family tradition of long standing. She has a special understanding of the challenges caregivers face in caring for people with Alzheimer's. For many years, Paula cared for her mother and grandmother in her home while raising two daughters and maintaining her career in nursing and health care management. Her personal and professional experience adds depth to many chapters of this book. Paula is active in several prominent professional organizations—SCCM, ENA, AACN, NFNA—and holds both local and national board positions. Paula is a native Oregonian and lives with her husband in Portland.

Susan Imke is a certified gerontological nurse practitioner with more than 20 years experience working with patients who have Parkinson disease and family caregivers. Originally certified as a family nurse practitioner, her focus shifted to elder care in the 1980s when she was appointed Associate Director of the Texas Tech Alzheimer Center in Lubbock, and later recruited to practice with a leading movement-disorder specialist, Abraham Lieberman, at the Barrow Neurological Institute in Pheonix. Susan is the CEO of Senior Health Solutions, a geriatric consulting practice, helping families living with chronic illnesses to navigate a complex health care system and maximize the functional abilities of the individual with neurological impairment. She serves on the Center of Excellence Review Board for the National Parkinson Foundation and on the Board of Directors for The Parkinson Alliance in Princeton, NJ. Susan lives with her husband in Fort Worth, Texas, and is the down-the-street caregiver for her 90-year-old father, who is recently widowed and has Parkinson disease.

Our Mission

CareTrust Publications is committed to providing high-quality, user-friendly information to those who face their own illness or the responsibilities of caring for friends, family, or clients.

Dedication

This book is dedicated to the memory of Pope John Paul II, whose willingness to share his Parkinson journey openly with the world provided encouragement and hope to all people who live with Parkinson disease.

Dear Caregiver,

Caring for someone with a chronic illness like Parkinson disease can be deeply satisfying as well as uniquely challenging. Partners, family, and friends can be drawn more closely together when they meet those challenges. Yet, caregiving can also be physically and emotionally exhausting, especially for the person who is the primary caregiver.

The Comfort of Home™ for Parkinson Disease: A Guide for Caregivers offers basic yet complete answers to your questions about caregiving. Although the book discusses issues specific to caring for someone with PD, it also contains valuable information that will be of help to any caregiver. This guide to in-home care uses current best practices in the areas it covers. It offers practical tips for many activities of daily living and the more complicated and stressful situations a caregiver may face. It also includes a wide-ranging list of resources for further reading and study.

The *Guide* has three parts:

Part One, Getting Ready, reviews caregiving options and discusses the medical decisions you may encounter. It shows how to set up a home in a safe and comfortable way for the person whose needs are changing and abilities are declining. Perhaps most important, it teaches you how to communicate better with doctors, nurses, aides, and pharmacists to get the services you need.

Part Two, Day by Day, guides you through every aspect of daily care. This may be as basic as bathing or helping someone transfer from a chair to a bed, or as daring as traveling with a person whose health is declining.

Part Three, Additional Resources, provides a list of informative and inspirational publications and a glossary of terms used to describe and explain symptoms or conditions.

Because a picture is worth a thousand words, we frequently use illustrations throughout the guide. And we include information that will guide you to organizations that will be invaluable in helping you provide care.

Being a caregiver is not for the timid and fearful. However, having as much knowledge as possible will help you overcome your fears. With this guide in hand, you will understand what help is needed and learn where to find it or how to provide it yourself.

Warm regards,

Maria & Paula

Maria and Paula

Acknowledgments

The procedures described in this *Guide* are based on research and consultation with experts in the fields of nursing, medicine, design, and law. The authors thank the innumerable professionals and caregivers who assisted in the development of this book.

This volume would not have been possible without the support of the American Parkinson Disease Association, the European Parkinson's Disease Association, and the National Parkinson Foundation. These organizations very generously allowed us access to their information, which details the most recent treatment and approaches to living with Parkinson disease. Readers can get more information on many of the subjects described in this *Guide* free of charge through the brochures available from these organizations:

American Parkinson Disease Association (APDA)
www.apadaparkinson.org

European Parkinson's Disease Association (EPDA)
www.epda.eu.com

National Parkinson Foundation (NPF)
www.parkinson.org

Special thanks go to the following people who shared their expertise in Parkinson disease. They kindly took the time to review the text and offered comments, suggestions, and support.

Carla Cothran, RN

Kathrynne Holden, MS, RD

Peter Hoogendoorn
Past President
Parkinson Patientien Vereniging

Lyndsey Isaacs
Wife of Tom Isaacs
Person with Parkinson Disease
United Kingdom

Susanna Lindvall
Vice Chair
Swedish Parkinson's Association

We are especially grateful to the following reviewers who made comments on sections of *The Comfort of Home*™ during its development:

Judy Alleman, RN, MN
CNS, Gerontology,
Professor, Mental Health Nursing,
Clark College

Mary J. Amdall-Thompson, RN, MS
Program Executive-Professional Services,
Oregon Board of Nursing

Sonya Beebe, RN
Executive Director,
Elder Abode, Lincoln City, Oregon

Brad Bowman, MD
CEO, WellMed, Inc.

Beth Boyd-Roberts, PT
Physical Therapy–In-Patient Supervisor

Karen Foley, OTR
Director, Regional Rehabilitation Services

Ruth Freeman, CNA
Caregiver

Kay B. Girsberger, RD

Esther King, RN, MN
Professor of Nursing, Clark College

Toni Lonning, MSW, LCSW
Social Worker/Care Manager

Betty McCallum, RN, BSN

Sylvia McSkimming, PhD, RD
Executive Director,
Supportive Care of the Dying:
A Coalition for Compassionate Care

James L. Meyer, AIA

Donald E. Nielsen, AIA

Northwest Parish Nurses Board of Directors

Cheryl Olson, RN, MBA
Director of Clinical Operations,
Home Services

Pamela Pauli, RN, MN

David L. Sanders, AIA
President, HPD Cambridge

Annette Stixrud, RN, MS
Program Director,
Northwest Parish Nurse Ministries

James Sturgis
Executive Director, Rose Villa, Inc.

Diane Welch, RN, MN
Associate Professor of Nursing
Linfield College

We thank them for their significant contributions, without which the quality and comprehensiveness of this *Guide* would not have been possible.

To Our Readers

Being told that the person in your care has Parkinson disease can be overwhelming for both of you. You may feel many mixed emotions, ranging from disbelief and denial to fear, anxiety, and sadness. At the same time, you may be relieved that a reason has finally been given for the person's problems.

Parkinson disease is a very individual condition and affects everyone differently. If someone you know or someone in your family has had Parkinson disease, do not assume that the person in your care will have the same symptoms or problems. Learn to recognize the symptoms in the person in your care and share any observations with the doctor and health care team.

How the individual and the family weather the storm depends on how healthy the relationships were before the disease began. The outcome depends on how severe the condition is and on the personalities of the individual and other family members. It will also depend on how close the family is, how much they rely on one another, and their cultural background.

One of the best ways to deal with any fears or worries about Parkinson disease is to find out as much as you can about the condition. Besides talking to your health care team, there are books and information on the Internet that can be useful sources of information. There are also dozens of Web sites hosted by Parkinson disease organizations. (See *Parkinson Disease and Caregiver Organizations* as well as *Resources* sections at the end of every chapter for contact and publication information.) The Glossary in this *Guide* features a list of common PD terms and symptoms (p. 265). Parkinson disease support groups in your local community are especially helpful as a place to learn from people who are sharing the same experiences.

The Comfort of Home™ for Parkinson Disease: A Guide for Caregivers is not meant to replace medical care but to add to the medical advice and services you receive from health care professionals. You should seek professional medical advice from a health care provider. This book is only a guide; follow your common sense and good judgment.

Neither the authors nor the publisher are engaged in rendering legal, accounting, or other professional advice. Seek the services of a competent professional if legal, architectural, or other expert assistance is required. The *Guide* does not represent Americans with Disabilities Act compliance.

Every effort has been made at the time of publication to provide accurate names, addresses, and phone numbers in the resource sections at the ends of chapters. The resources listed are those that benefit readers nationally. For this reason we have not included many local groups that offer valuable assistance. Failure to include an organization does not mean that it does not provide a valuable service. On the other hand, inclusion does not imply an endorsement. The authors and publisher do not warrant or guarantee any of the products described in this book and did not perform any independent analysis of the products described.

Throughout the book, we use "he" and "she" interchangeably when referring to the caregiver and the person being cared for.

ATTENTION NONPROFIT ORGANIZATIONS, CORPORATIONS, AND PROFESSIONAL ORGANIZATIONS: *The Comfort of Home™ for Parkinson Disease* is available at special quantity discounts for bulk purchases for gifts, fundraising, or educational training purposes. Special books, book excerpts, or booklets can also be created to fit specific needs. For details, write to CareTrust Publications LLC, P.O. Box 10283, Portland, Oregon 97296-0283, or call 1-800-565-1533.

Praise for *The Comfort of Home*™ Caregiver Guides

"This is an invaluable addition to bibliographies for the home caregiver. Hospital libraries will want to have a copy on hand for physicians, nurses, social workers, chaplains, and any staff dealing with MS patients and their caregivers. Highly recommended for all public libraries and consumer health collections."
—*Library Journal*

"A well-organized format with critical information and resources at your fingertips . . . educates the reader about the many issues that stand before people living with chronic conditions and provides answers and avenues for getting the best care possible."
—MSWorld, Inc. www.msworld.org

"A masterful job of presenting the multiple aspects of caregiving in a format that is both comprehensive and reader-friendly . . . important focus on physical aspects of giving care."
—Parkinson Report

"Almost any issue or question or need for resolution is most likely spoken of somewhere within the pages of this guide."
—*American Journal of Alzheimer's Disease*

"Physicians, family practitioners and geriatricians, and hospital social workers should be familiar with the book and recommend it to families of the elderly."
—Reviewers Choice, Home Care University

"An excellent guide on caregiving in the home. Home health professionals will find it to be a useful tool in teaching family caregivers."
—Five Star Rating, *Doody's Health Sciences Review Journal*

"Overall a beautifully designed book with very useful, practical information for caregivers."
—Judges from the Benjamin Franklin Awards

"Noteable here are the specifics. Where others focus on psychology alone, this gets down to the nitty gritty."
—*The Midwest Book Review*

"We use *The Comfort of Home*™ for the foundational text in our 40-hour Caregiver training. I believe it is the best on the market."
—Linda Young, Project Manager, College of the Desert

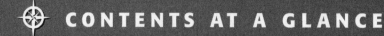

CONTENTS AT A GLANCE

Part Three   *Additional Resources*

Part One: Getting Ready

What Is Parkinson Disease?

What Is Parkinson Disease?

*P*arkinson disease (PD) is a chronic (ongoing) and slowly progressive neurological (involving the nervous system) condition. It is medically classified as a movement disorder, resulting from the depletion of a neurotransmitter (chemical messenger) called dopamine, produced in the mid-brain region known as the substantia nigra (black substance). The cause of this accelerated dopamine depletion is unknown, although genetic predisposition and environmental toxins may play a role. More detailed information on the anatomy and physiology of PD is available in numerous PD publications listed at the end of this chapter.

Approximately 1.2 million people in the United States have Parkinson disease, with possibly four million people diagnosed worldwide. Most people are diagnosed with PD in their 50's and 60's, but approximately 15% are diagnosed prior to age 50. Diagnosis prior to age 40 is categorized as young-onset PD.

While there is currently no cure for Parkinson disease, it is important to note that PD is not a condition that shortens life expectancy. The goals of medical treatment and allied health therapies are to minimize symptoms and maximize functional abilities in people living with Parkinson disease.

Early Detection of Parkinson Disease

Initially, mild symptoms of PD can come and go, and may be falsely attributed to normal aging. A unilateral (one-sided) tremor (shaking) of the hand is the most commonly noticed first symptom. About 25% of patients do not have a tremor, but may just feel very slow moving, easily fatigued, or aware of a change in gait (walk) and balance. Some people experience signs of anxiety or depression, or even chronic pain early in the illness. Family members may be first to observe some of these symptoms, or notice diminished facial expression, lowered voice volume, or decreased hand coordination performing routine tasks. Lack of arm swing on the affected side, and small, cramped handwriting (micrographia) are also common early signs.

Hallmark signs of Parkinson disease include:

- Unilateral resting tremor (when limb is not in motion)

- Bradykinesia (slowness of movement beyond that of normal aging)

- Rigidity (stiffness in limbs beyond that of normal aging)

- Postural instability (balance impairment, tendency to fall backward)

Two of the first three hallmark signs of PD should be detected before a diagnosis of Parkinson disease can be presumed. Because there are no lab tests or diagnostic procedures to confirm PD, it is said to be a *clinical diagnosis*, meaning it is based solely on the examination and observations of a trained physician. Both patients and family caregivers find this frustrating, leaving them to sometimes question whether the diagnosis is accurate. (See Resources at the end of this chapter for more detailed information.)

Caregivers might watch for additional symptoms that can appear early in the course of the disease or may become more apparent over time:

- Difficulty arising from a chair and changing position in bed

- Decreased fine-motor coordination (affects hand and finger mobility)

- Dysarthria (low voice volume or muffled speech)
- Shuffling gait or a tendency to drag one foot slightly when walking
- Reduced eye blinking and frequency of swallowing
- Anxiety and depression, difficulty concentrating
- Seborrhea (dandruff due to overproductive oil glands)
- Constipation
- Low blood pressure
- Sleep disorders

Unilateral symptoms may become bilateral (affecting both sides of the body) over time, although the primary side of involvement will always have more pronounced symptoms.

NOTE Symptoms vary significantly from one person to another and within the same person from day to day and at varying times of the day. Caregivers should be aware of these functional fluctuations in response to medication effects, or perhaps in response to varying stress or activity levels. Your person with Parkinson disease will need your help sometimes, but not at others. Encourage the person in your care to remain as independent as possible.

Tip Approximately 15% of persons initially diagnosed with PD do not have classical idiopathic (cause unknown) Parkinson disease, but rather one of several "look alike" syndromes. If symptoms are not responding to antiparkinson medications or the progression of the disease seems more rapid than is typical, it is important to get a second opinion to confirm or revise the diagnosis from a neurologist who has completed a fellowship in movement disorders.

> **NOTE** The physical ability of the person with PD changes through-out the day in response to antiparkinson medication. The person may not be able to dress and eat as well at certain times. He or she will need help sometimes and not at others. Let the person in your care remain as independent as possible.

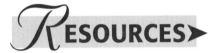

RESOURCES

For more information on the material presented in this chapter and free brochures on all topics related to Parkinson disease, contact:

American Parkinson Disease Association (APDA)
(800) 223-2732
www.apdaparkinson.org

European Parkinson's Disease Association (EPDA)
www.epda.eu.com

National Parkinson Foundation (NPF)
(800) 327-4545
www.parkinson.org

Books

Defying Despair: How One Man Is Winning His Battle with Young Onset Parkinson's Disease by Anthony Scelta, Jr., Myson Publishing, 2004.

Living with Parkinson's Disease by Bridget McCall, Sheldon Press, 2006.

Managing Parkinson's Disease – a series of educational booklets plus an exercise CD.
Available from Novartis Pharmaceuticals, 2005, www.stepkit.net

Parkinson's Disease. A Guide for Patient and Family
by Roger Duvoisin, Jacob Sage.

Parkinson's Disease: Questions and Answers, Third Edition by Robert Hauser and Theresa Zesiewicz, Merit Publishing, 2000.
Provided to health professionals and families by Novartis Pharmaceuticals

Shaking Up Parkinson Disease: Fighting Like a Tiger, Thinking Like a Fox by Abraham Lieberman, MD, Jones and Bartlett Publishers, 2002.

300 Tips for Making Life with Parkinson's Easier
by Shelley Peterman Schwarz, Demos Publishing.

Understanding Parkinson's Disease: A Self-Help Guide
by David Cram.

What Your Doctor May Not Tell You About Parkinson's Disease: A Holistic Program for Optimal Wellness
by Jill Marjama-Lyons, M.D. and Mary J. Shomon, Warner Books, 2003.

PD Medications and Wearing-Off

PD Medications and Wearing-Off

Most antiparkinson medications are intended to replenish, mimic, or enhance the natural dopamine that is lacking in the brain of the person with Parkinson disease. Drugs that alter dopamine levels are referred to as dopaminergic agents, which help alleviate muscle rigidity, reduce tremor, and improve speed and coordination of movement.

- Levodopa (Sinemet, Carbi/Levo *are common brand names) is still the "gold standard" of antiparkinson therapy. Levodopa is converted by brain cells into dopamine. This medication works well for many years, but over time can cause dyskinesias (involuntary writhing movements, usually when medication is at peak effect) and other troublesome side effects.*

- Dopamine agonists (Mirapex, Requip, and Permax *are common brand names) do not have to be converted into dopamine, but mimic its effects by acting directly on dopamine receptors in the brain. Dopamine agonists are now recommended as first-line prescription drug therapy to treat PD. These medications may adequately control PD symptoms for 2–4 years before levodopa therapy is required.*

- COMT (catechol-O-methyl-transferase) inhibitors (Comtan, Stalevo, Tasmar) *are taken with each dose of levodopa to extend duration of action.*

- Amantadine *is an antiviral agent that helps control Parkinson symptoms and dyskinesias caused by levodopa.*

- Anticholinergic *medications* (Artane, Benedryl, Cogentin) *can help control tremors but may worsen dry eyes, constipation, bladder problems, and glaucoma.*

- Antidepressants and antianxiety *medications can help manage mood disorders, which are common in PD.*

More detailed information regarding medications to treat symptoms of Parkinson disease is available from the Web sites and patient education publications available from the American Parkinson Disease Association and the National Parkinson Foundation.

What Is Wearing-Off?

Wearing-off is when Parkinson symptoms begin to reappear or become noticeably worse before it is time to take the next scheduled dose of medication. As wearing-off becomes more obvious, it may be harder to control the time when levodopa results in a good response ("on" time) and the time when there is a poor response to levodopa ("off" time).

It is important to be aware of the changes in symptoms that may indicate wearing-off. In this way, it may be possible to adjust therapy to provide better control of symptoms. As these changes take place, other unwanted drug-induced effects may also occur. These include involuntary movements such as dyskinesia (twisting, turning movements) or dystonia (abnormal positions and postures).

Tip

People come to their appointments at their "best," so doctors often don't recognize the signs of wearing-off. Be sure to mention to the doctor if symptoms have been returning before the next scheduled dose.

Common PD Terms

On-time is the when the levodopa or other Parkinson medication is having a benefit, and the parkinsonian symptoms are generally well controlled.

Off-time is when the PD medication is no longer working well for the parkinsonian symptoms. This may result in symptoms such as slowness, stiffness or tremor, and sometimes a total immobility (akinesia) or partial immobility (bradykinesia).

On-off phenomenon refers to sudden, sometimes unpredictable, changes in your symptoms. These changes vary from mobility (usually with dyskinesia) to immobility, due to the return of parkinsonian symptoms. There doesn't seem to be a connection between these sudden changes and the timing of the medication.

Wearing-off is when the improvement gained from a dose of levodopa medication gradually weakens and does not last until the next scheduled dose is due or begins to work. (This feeling often has been compared to a car running out of fuel.) You may feel that the person in your care needs the next dose of medication sooner.

Delayed on is when there is an increased delay between taking the levodopa medication and feeling its benefits. This may be more common with controlled-release preparations of levodopa, which take time to dissolve in the stomach, enter the bloodstream, and travel into the brain in sufficient quantities to replace the missing dopamine.

Freezing episodes are sudden, brief periods of immobility that last from seconds to minutes. The person in your care may feel "stuck to the spot," as if glued to the floor. Freezing most often occurs when trying to start walking, while turning in confined spaces, or when going through doorways.

Dyskinesia describes the abnormal, twisting, turning, "dancelike" movements that follow prolonged treatment with levodopa preparations. These involuntary movements are often associated with the peak effects of levodopa and usually appear about the same time as wearing-off.

Dystonia involves sustained involuntary muscle contractions that result in abnormal positions or postures, most frequently in the foot. Dystonia can occur in "on" periods (when the person is usually mobile) or in "off" periods, or both. Early morning dystonia refers to muscle cramping occurring in the early morning hours prior to taking the first morning dose of medication. This is usually seen as downward curling of the toes.

Tip

Caregivers must know that early-morning toe cramping is caused by low levels of dopamine. Beware of podiatrists who diagnose the problem as hammer toes and recommend needless surgery.

Common Symptoms of Wearing-Off

As caregiver, watch for symptoms that may indicate the person in your care is experiencing wearing-off. Note whether the symptoms tend to worsen two or more hours after the last dose of levodopa medication, and whether they improve after the next levodopa dose takes effect.

Motor Symptoms

Motor symptoms relate to movement and mobility. These include—

- Tremor—shakiness or trembling in the hands, arms, legs, jaw, and face. Some people feel an internal tremor (trembling inside) even though this may not be visible.

- Rigidity—stiffness in the muscles causing movements to become more uncomfortable.

Typical pattern of wearing-off during the day.

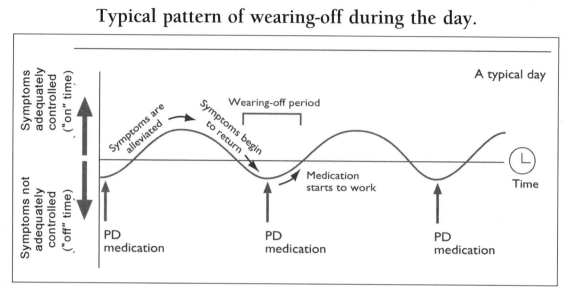

Reprinted with permission of the European Parkinson's Disease Association.

- Slowness of movement (bradykinesia)—movements become slow and hesitant and it takes more time to perform daily activities or the person may be temporarily unable to perform activities at all.

Non-motor Symptoms

Some symptoms that affect thoughts, feelings, sensations, and sense of well-being:

- anxiety, depression, or irritability
- slowness of thinking or memory problems
- tingling
- restlessness
- pain
- fatigue
- sweating
- extreme salivation

- changing body temperature
- constipation

> **NOTE** Simply put, wearing-off is when the benefits of levodopa taper off and symptoms reoccur before the next scheduled dose is due.

Treatment of Wearing-Off

If the person in your care is experiencing symptoms of wearing-off, the doctor will probably explore a range of treatments:

- evaluating the daily routine and adjusting the medication's timing and dose
- changing the current therapy in order to increase the person's "on time" and decrease the "off time" and reduce any side effects
- using additional medications or combinations of medications to provide enough symptom control without side effects

> **NOTE** It should be noted, however, that most persons with PD prefer being "on" with dyskinesia rather than being "off."

> **NOTE** Involuntary movements, known as dyskinesia, are a side effect of PD medication, particularly levodopa. Similar to wearing-off, dyskinesia often appears 2 to 3 years after the start of levodopa therapy. If the person in your care does experience dyskinesia, remember to record it in the diary. This will help the doctor adjust the medication.

Tracking Motor Fluctuations or "On/Off Tracking"

To help decide if the person in your care is having wearing-off, the doctor sometimes uses a questionnaire called the Unified Parkinson Disease Rating Scale (UPDRS) or a simplified reporting card such as the one shown on page 18.

The patient card may also help the doctor be aware of wearing-off symptoms, both motor and non-motor. The doctor can then talk to you about these symptoms, what impact they may have on the person's daily life, and the best way to manage them.

KEEP A DIARY

Work with the specialist team to find the best way to become aware of and manage PD symptoms. Provide them with an exact description of daily medication, how the person reacts to these medications, and possible side effects. It will help in choosing the treatment options if you can describe the pattern of symptoms from day to day and even hour to hour.

Keeping a Diary

It is not always easy to know which wearing-off symptoms a person is having. One way is to keep a diary of when medication is taken, how long the benefits last, and possible side effects. Diary forms are often available from movement disorder offices or national PD organizations. The diary could be kept for a week or so, just before the next doctor's appointment. The doctors may want to keep a copy of the diary in the medical record.

The types of information to put in a diary include

- the times of day when the Parkinson medications are taken

- the times of day when there is good symptom control

- which symptoms come back during the day and when

- which symptoms appear at night

- any effects the person may have, such as dyskinesia, and their relation to when the person takes the medication

Note the timing of meals and snacks and whether this affects symptom control. To help decide if this is wearing-off, it may be useful to rate each of the Parkinson symptoms, which symptoms are the worst, and how they affect the daily life of the person in your care.

Some people rate their symptoms by number, as we have shown in the Wearing-Off Question Card. Other people use words to describe their symptoms (see list on p. 14). Use a scale that you and the care receiver find the easiest to use and that has meaning for both.

Tip

Doctors may focus on your motor symptoms only, but let them know about bothersome anxiety and fatigue. This may also be a sign that the medication is wearing-off.

Wearing-Off Question Card

Please check in **Column A** any symptoms that you currently experience in your normal day. Please also check the box in **Column B** if this symptom usually improves or disappears after you take your next dose of your Parkinson's medication.

	COLUMN A Experience symptoms	COLUMN B Usually improves after my next dose
1. Slowness of movement (bradykinesia)	☐	☐
2. Tremors	☐	☐
3. Feeling of internal tremors	☐	☐
4. Decreased manual dexterity	☐	☐
5. Inability to move (akinesia) in the early morning	☐	☐
6. Sudden muscle spasms (dystonia)	☐	☐
7. "Pins and needles" feeling (parasthesia)	☐	☐
8. Muscle pain	☐	☐
9. Voice softness	☐	☐

Source: Stacy, M. (2003). End of dose wearing-off in Parkinson's disease: Sensitivity comparison of a patient survey versus a programmed investigator evaluation. *European Journal of Neurology,* (Suppl. 10), 1:20.

> **Tip** Sometimes a person with PD becomes withdrawn from friends because of embarrassment due to tremors, drooling, or difficulty eating or moving. If this happens, ask the doctor to treat the symptoms or refer the person for physical therapy, occupational therapy, or counseling.

Pointers for Using Parkinson Medications Effectively

It is essential that patients and caregivers become knowledgeable about the medications used to treat Parkinson disease. Medical research has provided numerous medications that used alone, or more often in careful combination, can provide significant relief of PD symptoms. Intelligent use of these medications can greatly enhance the person in your care's quality of life.

The following tips are especially noteworthy in learning to use the antiparkinson medications:

- There is a tremendous variability of PD symptoms and response to treatment from one individual to another.

- Medication choices and doses must be tailored for an individual patient's needs at a specific point in time. The doctor and patient must work closely as a team to make needed adjustments.

- The timing of medication doses is almost as important as what medications are taken. The reason timing is so crucial is discussed in the next chapter (see Tracking Motor Fluctuations or "On/Off Tracking," p. 16).

- *Any* medication may cause unwanted side effects during the course of therapy. Side effects must be discussed with the physician so doses can be adjusted or discontinued.

- Most patients are optimally managed on a combination of medications instead of continuing to increase the amount of levodopa as solo therapy.

- Allied health services such as physical therapy, occupational therapy, speech therapy, and counseling are invaluable adjunct treatments in maintaining good motor function.

The ultimate goal of comprehensive therapy is to maximize current physical and mental function while maintaining options for a healthy future.

Tip

Caregivers might watch for clues that their person with PD needs help monitoring medications. Most patients manage their own medication doses and timing in the early years, but may need help along the way if confusion becomes a problem or awkward hand movements aren't compatible with pill bottle manipulations.

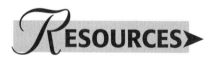 RESOURCES

For more information on the material presented in this chapter and free brochures on all topics related to Parkinson disease, contact:

American Parkinson Disease Association (APDA)
(800) 223-2732
www.apdaparkinson.org

European Parkinson's Disease Association (EPDA)
www.epda.eu.com

National Parkinson Foundation (NPF)
(800) 327-4545
www.parkinson.org

A Caregivers Guide to Giving Medications by Carol Heerema
Pearson PTR © 1999.

Using the Health Care Team Effectively

Using the Health Care Team Effectively

When you care for someone in the home, you must also manage that person's health care. This means choosing a good medical team, keeping costs down, arranging for surgery, and getting the best, least expensive medicines. It also means knowing what the insurance rules are and, most important, being an advocate (a supporter) for the person in your care.

Once the person in your care has been diagnosed with Parkinson disease, you will need to work with a team of health care specialists. They will help find the best way to manage symptoms. You may not need the support of every member of this team right away. The ones you see on a daily basis may change as treatment needs change.

NOTE As the caregiver, remember that you, the person in your care, and the person's family are key members of the team.

An Effective Team for Managing Parkinson Disease

The person in your care and his or her family are a central part of the team.

The **family doctor (or primary care physician)** is usually the first point of contact. You and the person in your care will probably see this doctor most often over the years. The primary care doctor looks after the person's general health and helps coordinate care with other health care professionals.

Neurologists have specialized knowledge of Parkinson disease. Visits will be occasional and referral is normally from the primary care physician. Not all neurologists are expert in PD management. It may be wise to ask for a referral to a movement disorders specialist.

You may see a **nurse practitioner** or **physician assistant** sometimes instead of a doctor.

The **pharmacist** is another important part of your team. Try to use the same pharmacy all the time so there is a record of all medications being taken. The pharmacist can give you advice about drug treatments and ensure that over-the-counter medications and vitamin supplements do not interact with prescription drugs.

The **physical therapist** (or **physiotherapist** as he or she is called in Europe) can look into problems with mobility (ability to move around), balance, and posture. Because PD affects movement control, exercise plays an important role in helping people with PD have a healthy lifestyle. A physical therapist can also advise on exercise and on overcoming symptoms so that it doesn't have as much impact on the person's daily routine.

Occupational therapists can help with planning the person's day. They can advise you and the person in your care about balancing work, relaxation, and leisure activities. (Having Parkinson disease does not mean that a person has to give up his or her job.)

A **counselor** can provide individual or family counseling. The difficulties caused by PD can often be accompanied by feelings of sadness and depression. A counselor can help everyone adjust to the changes.

Speech and language therapists can help the person speak more clearly and with problems such as speaking too softly. They can also help with swallowing problems (📖 see *Resources*).

A **registered dietician** can advise on planning a healthful diet and maintaining the right weight. If there are problems with weight loss (or gain) or constipation, the doctor may refer the person to a dietician. Dietary advice may also benefit treatment, because diet and when you eat can affect how medications work.

A **psychologist** may provide advice and counseling if the person is having difficulty coping with the disease emotionally or with such things as memory problems.

A **psychiatrist** is an expert in mental health problems who can help with problems such as depression, anxiety, and disturbances in thinking and perception. These symptoms may require specialized treatment.

A **social worker** may provide nonmedical assistance. This might include help with the general management of Parkinson disease, financial advice, and respite care. A social worker will be able to access available community resources and find the right financial assistance program for you.

> **NOTE** Don't be afraid to ask the family doctor for a referral to a specialist. A neurologist will have specialized knowledge on how best to treat Parkinson disease.

Choosing a Doctor

Both the APDA and NPF can recommend names of neurologists who specialize in PD. Think about using doctors who are allied with medical schools or movement disorder treatment centers. They tend to have the most up-to-date information and access to clinical trials.

- Make sure the doctor is board certified in his or her specialty.

- If the person in your care is enrolled in a managed care plan, ask if the doctor is planning to continue being an approved provider.

- You can contact more than one doctor (for a second opinion). If you are enrolled in Medicare Supplementary Medical Insurance (Part B), Medicare will pay for a second opinion in the same way it pays for other services.

Regular Doctor Visits

Regular visits to the doctor are important for ensuring that the person in your care is getting the best medical attention possible. The person can tell the doctor how he or she is feeling about the condition and the treatment and get answers to any questions. Report the results of any drug regimen to the doctor. Tell the doctor if there is something you don't understand. Learn the terms the doctor uses, so that it will be easier to discuss treatments. (📖 See *Common PD Terms,* p. 12.)

When you visit any health care professional, bring a list of questions and concerns. Also bring a notebook to write down what you are told.

Try to build a good relationship with the health care team. Ask for the help you need to manage the symptoms of the person in your care.

You may want to ask the following questions:

- How soon will we see a noticeable improvement after medications have been started?

- Will there be any side effects?

- Does the person's diet or mealtimes have an effect on how well medications work?

- Should the person be taken to a Parkinson disease specialist?

- What other treatments are available?

> **NOTE** Not all problems are related to PD. Be on the lookout for other difficulties the person may be having. It is important not to overlook problems that may not be related to PD.

Caregivers may find it difficult or embarrassing to talk about some of the PD symptoms. Remember that the people on the team are experienced health care professionals, and they want to work with you to help resolve these problems.

Doctors and nurses may focus on physical diagnosis and ignore the emotional aspects of care. Sometimes they have little time to consider the spiritual aspects of healing. Although you should consult with professionals about the levels of therapy and support needed for the person in your care, you do not need to accept what they suggest or order. Keep asking questions until you thoroughly understand the diagnosis (what is wrong), treatment, and prognosis (likely outcome).

How to Share in Medical Decisions

Important medical decisions are the responsibility of the person in your care, the doctor, and the caregiver. Don't be afraid to take an active role and be an advocate for the person in your care.

Long-Range Considerations

- Find out how the person in your care feels about treatments that prolong life. Respect those views.

- Help the person receiving care set up an advance directive and power of attorney for health care.

- Share decisions with the doctor and the care receiver. Accept responsibility for the treatment and its outcomes.

The Doctor–Patient–Caregiver Relationship

- Be aware that doctors must see more patients every day than they once did.

- Some doctors have financial reasons for doing too much or too little for those in their care. Specialists are often the only ones with the training needed to treat a serious or chronic condition.

- If the relationship with the doctor becomes unfriendly, find a new doctor.

- Respect the doctor's time. You may need to have more than one visit to cover all issues.

- If Medicare is your payer, ask if the doctor accepts Medicare assignment. If not, the difference may have to be paid out of pocket.

People with PD, particularly those who are elderly, may be at greater risk for pneumonia. It is important to call the doctor when there is a fever lasting longer than a few days, a wet cough, pain when taking deep breaths, and shortness of breath. This may be pneumonia, which can be fatal for those whose systems are weakened.

Preparing for a Visit to the Doctor

- Be prepared to explain briefly the care receiver's and the family's medical history.

- Bring a list of questions in order of importance.

- Be prepared to ask for written information about the medical situation so you can better understand what the doctor is saying. It may help to bring a small tape recorder.

- Call the hospital's library or health resource center. Ask the librarian for help in looking up any questions the doctor has not answered.

 NOTE Be sure shots for tetanus, flu, and pneumonia are up to date. For those on Medicare, flu and pneumonia shots are covered.

At the Doctor's Office

- Clearly explain to the doctor what you hope and expect from treatment.

- If the doctor tells you to do something you know you can't do—such as give medication in the middle of the night—ask for another treatment and explain why.

- Insist on talking about the level of care you believe is right for the person in your care and that agrees with his or her wishes.

- Look into other options to tests, medications, and surgery.

- Ask why tests or treatments are needed and what the risks are.

- Look at all options, including "watchful waiting."(By federal law, an insurance company must let a doctor discuss all treatment options.)

- Trust your common sense. If you have doubts, get a second opinion.

Questions to Ask Before Agreeing to Tests, Medications, and Surgery

Before you begin discussing medical treatment with the doctor, explain that the person in your care does not want any unnecessary tests or treatments. Then ask these questions:

- Why is this test needed?

- How long will it take? How soon will we see the results?

- Is it accurate?

- Is it painful?

- Are there risks in taking the test? Do the benefits outweigh the risks?

- How long after treatment will side effects occur and how long will they last?

- Are X rays necessary?

- Will the doctor review the test report with me and explain the details?

- Can a copy of the report be taken home? (If you have concerns, talk to the specialist who produced the report.)

- If a test is positive, what action should be taken?

- Is the condition going to worsen slowly or rapidly?

- What could happen if the test is not done?

- How much does the test cost and is there a less expensive one?

Questions to Ask the Doctor About Medications

You will need to work with the doctor to find the right balance of medications to manage the symptoms of the disease effectively. Treatment is usually started with low doses of a drug. The dose is then increased slowly, one step at a time, until the symptoms are under control.

The doctor will recommend a certain treatment for specific symptoms. Not everyone will receive the same medications. In the very early stages of the disease the person in your care may not need any medication at all.

The dose and timing of medications may need to be changed over time as symptoms change (or side effects occur). A combination of different medications is often required to provide the most effective symptom control.

No matter which medication is taken, it is important that you understand the following:

- How many or how much medication should the person in your care take?

- How the medication should be taken (for example, with food or between meals, with milk or water, etc.)?

- What other types of medication should not be used with the medication already being taken?

- Always discuss any side effects with the doctor.

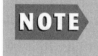 Avoid starting the person on a new medication when you will not be able to get to the doctor or other health care professional, such as before going on vacation.

Tip

Recent legislation regarding prescription drug insurance (Medicare Part D) in the U.S. has significantly reduced monthly medication costs for most enrollees. If the person in your care is eligible for coverage, ask your pharmacist to advise which plans provide the best coverage for the person's current prescriptions.

If he is eligible for Medicare Part D, most pharmacies will accept the same co-pay (for instance, $5 for generic [non-brand name] prescription for a 30-day supply). If the person is under age 65 and not eligible for Medicare benefits, then it pays to shop around locally or go online to compare prices from retail pharmacies. Discount warehouse stores such as Sam's Club and Costco often have lower prices than many independent pharmacies. In some cases, mail-ordering prescriptions may offer cost savings. If you value the more personalized services of a neighborhood pharmacist, it is wise to weigh convenience and access to the pharmacist as well as price when choosing a pharmacy.

Questions to Ask the Pharmacist

- Is there a generic drug that is the equivalent strength to the prescribed brand name drug that costs less per month?

- Reviewing the list of medications taken, are there possible negative interactions or potential side effects to watch for?

- Is the care receiver taking any nutritional supplements or other non-prescription medications that might have harmful side effects when combined with the prescription meds?

- Does the pharmacy have a computer program that will alert them to potential drug–drug interactions or drug–food interactions?

- Can the person taking this medication smoke or drink alcohol in moderation while using this drug? Is it OK for him to drive?

- When a single medication is expensive and not on the individual's prescription drug plan, can the pharmacist help with getting assistance from the pharmaceutical manufacturer or other sources to cover part of the cost?

- Is the person in your care taking any medications that should not be stopped abruptly, but rather tapered off if discontinued?

- Will the pharmacy contact the doctor to request medication changes or are you expected to be the communication link with the doctor?

- Will they substitute easy-open caps on pill vials for the clumsy child-proof tops?

Tip
Pharmacists often place numerous caution stickers on Rx bottles. Some risks are real, some *very* unlikely. Learn enough about the Parkinson medications to know which is which, and request that the pharmacist resist being overly cautious.

Tip
MEDICAL ALERT
A person with PD who is mobile should carry a card that lists all medications he or she is currently taking.

Surgical Therapy for Parkinson Disease

Neurosurgical procedures are now available and covered by insurers to treat some symptoms of Parkinson disease that no longer respond well to medication therapy alone.

Deep brain stimulation (DBS) is the most commonly chosen surgery. DBS involves placing a lead (thin wire), deep into the mid-brain. This lead is attached to a *neurostimulator* that is implanted in the chest wall. The neurostimulator is turned on and off by a magnetic device, much like a pacemaker for the heart. Deep brain stimulation is an effective treatment option for moderate to severe PD symptoms.

Other surgeries used to treat PD include thalamotomy, pallidotomy, and subthalamotomy. Of these, pallidotomy and DBS have produced the best results to date in treating PD. Patients who have surgery to help control Parkinson symptoms typically still require reduced doses of antiparkinson medication.

Pallidotomy is a technique in which a heated probe is inserted into the brain to precisely destroy a small area of brain cells in the region known as the globus pallidus. Pallidotomy can improve tremor, rigidity, bradykinesia, motor fluctuations, and in some cases, walking and balance.

There are advantages and disadvantages to pallidotomy and DBS:

Pallidotomy
- Permanently destroys a small area of brain cells
- Involves no implanted devices
- Should not be done bilaterally

Deep Brain Stimulation
- Does not destroy brain tissue
- Is reversible
- Can be done bilaterally
- Requires re-programming as symptoms change
- Involves the possibility of hardware malfunction

Both procedures involve a small risk for intracranial (within the skull) bleeding or strokes at the time of surgery. Neither procedure should be considered for a person with PD who also has dementia (marked confusion).

If you and the person in your care are considering surgery as a treatment to reduce PD symptoms:

- Consult with a neurologist who has completed a fellowship in movement disorders. This individual *should not* be the same neurosurgeon who will perform the elective surgery. Do not be shy about asking for the doctor's credentials.

- Do your homework. Learn about DBS and look into the hospitals you are considering. (NPF has a patient education booklet devoted to DBS.) Choose a neurosurgery center with an interdisciplinary team of healthcare professionals with the training, technology, and expertise required.

- Be prepared to invest a lot of time, energy, and travel for pre- and postoperative appointments. A significant number of postoperative visits are necessary during the first six months after surgery.

Questions to Ask About Surgery

Surgery is a serious step. Ask as many questions as you need before deciding to go ahead.

- Why does the person need the surgery?
- Will the surgery stop the problem or merely slow its progress?
- Are there other options?
- Can it be done on an outpatient basis (where the person is not admitted to the hospital)?
- What will happen if surgery is not done?
- Where will the surgery be done? When?
- Will the surgeon you spoke to do the surgery or will it be assigned to another doctor? (When going into

surgery, put the surgeon's name on the release form to ensure that the named surgeon is the one who does the operation.)

- How many surgeries of this type has the doctor performed? (Generally, the more times the surgeon has performed an operation, the higher the success rate will be.)

- What is the doctor's success rate with this type of surgery?

- What are the anesthesiologist's qualifications?

- What can go wrong?

- How much will it cost, and is it covered by insurance or Medicare?

- What other specialists should be asked for a second opinion? (Medicaid and Medicare usually pay for second opinions. Doctors expect people to go for a second opinion when surgery is needed, and they should help you find one.)

NOTE A second opinion should not come from a medical partner of the first-opinion doctor!

 MEDICAL RECORDS
To save costs, have all medical records and tests sent to the second doctor. Also, if possible, bring the important ones with you.

NOTE Even the experts don't always agree about the best treatment. The final decision is yours.

Alternative Treatments

Traditional and alternative medical providers want everyone to have a healthy lifestyle. If ill health is caused by stress, medications may provide only short-term relief. When stress is the cause, the reason for the stress should be looked into. However, if you are thinking of trying alternative health care, ask the same questions you would ask any medical specialist. Follow these guidelines:

- Be on guard against anyone who says to stop seeing a conventional (regular) doctor or to stop taking prescribed medicine.

- Meditate or exercise regularly to help reduce the need for prescription drugs.

- Remember, many insurance companies do not cover alternative medical practitioners.

Mental Health Treatment

Emotional changes are very common in PD. Common disorders include depression and anxiety, and unusual symptoms such as loss of impulse control and increased emotions.

All questions and problems should be openly spoken about with the doctor. (📖 See *Resources for NPF's, Mind, Mood, & Memory*).

> *Tip*
>
> Ignore unwanted behaviors by showing no emotion, not making eye contact, and not speaking of the behavior. Reward desired behavior with a touch or smile and a thank-you.

Strong emotions are a normal reaction to long-term illness. Psychological counseling and support groups are a very valuable source of help.

- For someone who is depressed and needs therapy, ask the primary care doctor for a referral to a therapist.

- Be aware that many people are embarrassed by mental health problems and are reluctant to seek care.

- For help deciding whether a person has the ability to make legal decisions, arrange for a psychiatrist's assessment.

Dental Care

Dental care is important for overall wellness. For low-cost dental programs, check with university dental schools (or the local Area Agency on Aging if the person in your care is older).

- Tell the dentist all the medications the person is taking before starting dental treatment.

- Go to a dentist who is familiar with Parkinson disease. (Ask your local chapter or support group for a list of names.)

- Find out how many visits will be needed each year to ensure good dental health.

- Ask about low-cost alternatives to the recommended treatment.

- Ask if X rays are really necessary.

- Find out the cost of dentures, but don't trust prices that seem too good to be true. Cheap dentures may not fit correctly.

- When seeking another opinion, have all medical records and tests sent to the second dentist.

Vision Care

Regular eye exams every two years (or yearly if the person in your care has diabetes) are important to see if lens corrections are needed and to detect any underlying eye diseases. Early detection of some treatable eye disorders can prevent blindness in the future.

Take the person in your care to see an eye specialist (ophthalmologist) who is licensed to diagnose disease as well as fit glasses. It may be helpful to get a referral to see a *neuroophthalmologist*, who is also knowledgeable about the visual problem in Parkinson disease. Some people with PD have problems with blurry vision or seeing double images. Some experience difficulties with visual contrast, seeing less well when objects are not "black and white." The visual problems in PD can be part of the illness, or may be caused by medications. Many people with PD don't suffer significant vision problems related to their PD.

Before going to the eye doctor:

- take a list of all prescription and non-prescription medications the person in your care is taking.

- tell the doctor if there is a family history of glaucoma, diabetes, or macular degeneration.

- ask for help finding adaptive devices (talking watches, reading aids, etc.) that might be useful for someone with low vision.

- contact your state or local Commission for the Blind for additional advice on adaptive products and aids to help with low vision.

Parkinson disease causes a reduction in automatic reflexes, which includes blinking of the eyes. This can lead to dry eye syndrome and sometimes more difficult conditions with the cornea (lens of the eye). Caregivers should apply artificial tears twice daily to remedy dry eyes. Have the person in your care lie down, put the drops in the inner corner with the eyelid closed, then have the person blink to distribute the saline. Never touch the dropper to the eye to prevent contamination.

Tip Be sure to buy the artificial tears (normal saline) product, not the "red out" formulas, which are more irritating to the eyes.

Sometimes persons with PD begin having visual hallucinations, which are almost always a side effect of the antiparkinson medications, not part of the disease itself. The caregiver will need to work with the doctor to reduce or discontinue the offending drug, or if it is essential to the person's motor function, to consider other medications to treat the hallucinations.

NOTE Danger signs to watch for are if the person sees changes in the color or size of an object when one eye is covered or when straight poles appear bent or wavy. Call an ophthalmologist without delay.

How to Watch Out for Someone's Best Interests in the Hospital

Someone who is the hospital is at greater risk than others, so be prepared to keep tabs on treatments, ask questions, and act as an advocate in the person's best interests.

- If the Patients' Bill of Rights isn't posted where it can be seen, ask for a copy.

- Only agree to procedures (tests, treatments, surgery, etc.) that make sense to you.

- If something is not being done and you think it should be, ask why.

- Be friendly and show respect to the hospital staff. They will probably respond better to you and the person in your care. Bad feelings between family members and staff may cause staff to avoid the person.

- Assist with grooming and care.

- Speak up if you notice doctors or nurses examining anyone without first washing their hands.

- After discharge, check all bills and ask about anything that isn't clear to you.

NOTE According to federal law, a hospital must release patients in a *safe manner* or else must keep them in the hospital. Letting a patient leave the hospital is unwise if the person has constant fever, infection or pain that cannot be controlled, confusion, disorientation (no sense of time or place), or is unable to take food and liquids by mouth. In some cases, however, it may be better for the person to be released because the noise and risk of catching other diseases while in the hospital may make it more difficult for the person to recover. If you plan to appeal a discharge, understand the rules of Medicare, Medicaid, the HMO, or the insurance plan.

When You Doubt the Time Is Right for Discharge

- State your doubts in a simple letter to the hospital's director or the health plan's medical director. (Rules are different from state to state.)

- Meet with the hospital's discharge planner.

- Ask if the hospital is following the usual policy for the condition.

Checklist **Coming Home from the Hospital**

✓ Assess the person's condition and needs.

✓ Understand the diagnosis (what is wrong) and prognosis (what will happen).

✓ Become part of the health care team (doctor, nurse, therapists) so you can learn how to provide care.

✓ Get complete written instructions from the doctor. If there is anything you don't understand, ASK QUESTIONS.

✓ Arrange follow-up care from the doctor.

✓ Develop a plan of care with the doctor. (📖 See **Setting Up a Plan of Care**, p. 103.)

✓ Meet with the hospital's social worker or discharge planner to determine home care benefits.

✓ Understand in-home assistance options. (📖 See **Getting In-Home Help**, p. 48.)

✓ Arrange for in-home help.

✓ Arrange physical, occupational, and speech therapy as needed.

✓ Find out if medicine is provided by the hospital to take home. If not, you will have to have prescriptions filled before you take the person home.

✓ Prepare the home. (📖 See **Preparing the Home**, p. 59.)

✓ Buy needed supplies; rent, borrow, or buy equipment such as wheelchairs, crutches, and walkers.

✓ Take home all personal items.

✓ Check with the hospital cashier for discharge payment requirements.

✓ Arrange transportation (an ambulance or van if your car will not do).

....

KEEP ASKING QUESTIONS UNTIL YOU ARE SATISFIED. Doctors and other health care professionals have medical know-how, but only you can explain symptoms. Report exactly, in as few words as possible, any unusual symptoms, changes in condition, and complaints the person has.

- Explain any special reasons that you think make it unwise to discharge the person.

- Ask if the usual hospital rules can be changed to cover this special case.

- Remember that anyone has the right to appeal a discharge.

- Get the doctor's help in the appeal, but understand that he or she may have different reasons for wanting to discharge the person.

NOTE Do not hesitate to call the hospital ombudsman, who is responsible for the patient's rights.

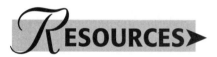

RESOURCES

For more information on the material presented in this chapter, and free brochures on all topics related to Parkinson disease, contact:

American Parkinson Disease Association (APDA)
(800) 223-2732
www.apdaparkinson.org

European Parkinson's Disease Association (EPDA)
www.epda.eu.com

National Parkinson Foundation (NPF)
(800) 327-4545
www.parkinson.org

Free or low-cost resources: local consumer health resource/information centers (check your local hospital system or phone book) and local health agencies or associations (American Heart Association, American Diabetes Association, Multiple Sclerosis Society, and others)

Doctor's Guide to the Internet—Patient Edition
www.pslgroup.com/PTGUIDE.HTM
Provides information for specific diseases and gives pointers to other Internet sites of medical information.

Go Ask Alice!
http://www.goaskalice.columbia.edu/about.html
Provides helpful information and lets you post health-related questions on the site.

The Health Resource, Inc.
933 Faulkner Street
Conway, AR 72034
(800) 949-0090; (501) 329-5272; Fax (501) 329-9489
www.thehealthresource.com
Provides clients with complete personal reports on their specific medical conditions. These reports contain treatments, both conventional and alternative, and information on current research, nutrition, self-help measures, specialists, and resource organizations. Reports on any noncancer condition are $295, or $395 for complex issues, and contain 50 to 100 pages. Reports on any cancer condition are $395 and contain 150 to 200 pages. Shipping is additional.

University of Washington
www.washington.edu/medical
A great storehouse of general health information on all topics.

Medications

Together Rx Access™ Card

A joint program by drug companies offering a free Prescription Savings Card for individuals and families who meet all four of the following requirements:

❏ Not eligible for Medicare
❏ Have no public or private prescription-drug coverage
❏ Household income equal to or less than:
—$30,000 for a single person
—$40,000 for a family of two
—$50,000 for a family of three
—$60,000 for a family of four
—$70,000 for a family of five

❏ Legal resident of the U.S. or Puerto Rico

Call 1-800-250-2839 to begin saving on your prescriptions. For the most current list of medicines and products, visit www.TogetherRxAccess.com

If you don't have access to the Internet, ask your local library to help you locate a Web site.

Getting In-Home Help

Getting In-Home Help

etting help with caregiving in the home involves the following options:

- *Use a Home Health Care Agency (Typical fee range: $50 to $150 per visit through a private agency)*

- *Hire someone privately (Typical fee range: $12 to $15 per hour—the cost of assistance is based on the category of professional)*

- *Perform all caregiving duties yourself.*

Use a Home Health Care Agency

Home Health Care Agencies are for-profit, nonprofit, or governmental. They ensure quality of care by providing personal care, skilled care, patient and caregiver instruction, and supervision. They usually provide certified nurse assistants (CNAs), sometimes called home health aides; registered nurses (RNs); licensed practical nurses (LPNs); physical therapists; occupational therapists; and speech therapists by training. (A doctor's order is required to obtain reimbursement for skilled-care nursing in the home.) These agencies help plan services and care that match the health, social, and financial needs of the client.

Definitions for Agencies

There are a number of terms to describe an agency's services. Study them carefully before looking into those in your area.

Accredited—Services have been reviewed by a nonprofit organization interested in quality home health care.

Bonded—The agency has paid a fixed dollar amount in order to be bonded. In the event of court action the bond pays the penalties. (Being bonded does not ensure good service.)

Certified—The agency has met federal standards for care and takes part in the Medicare program.

Certified Health Personnel—Those who work for the agency meet the standards of a licensing agency for the state.

Insurance Claims Honored—The agency will look into insurance benefits and accepts assignment of benefits (meaning the insurance company pays the agency directly).

Licensed—The agency has met the requirements to run its business (in those states that oversee home health care agencies).

Licensed Health Personnel—The people who work for the agency have passed the state licensing exam for that profession.

Screened—References have been checked; a criminal check may also have been made.

How to Pay for an Agency

Paying for care from an agency ranges from Medicare to private pay to long-term-care insurance to state and county programs.

Medicare

To be eligible for the Medicare home-health benefit, a person must basically be unable to leave the house (be homebound) and need periodic skilled care.

- Medicare pays the full cost of medically necessary home health visits by a Medicare-approved home health agency.

- Medicare will pay for some elderly care if the person qualifies for skilled care (expertise of a registered nurse) that is not considered maintenance.

- The person must be as unable to care for himself or herself as someone who would otherwise be in a nursing home.

 NOTE States vary on eligibility requirements, so check with your area Medicare office for local rules.

Private Pay

- If a person does not qualify for public funds, he or she must pay with long-term-care insurance or pay privately.

- Care management through Area Agencies on Aging may be free or offered on a sliding scale, based on a person's income.

What the Home Health Agency Will Do

- schedule an in-home visit

- carry out an assessment (by a registered nurse) to determine the level of care required

- look into insurance benefits and publicly funded benefits

- ask for an assignment of benefits

- ask you to sign a form to release of medical information

- ask you to agree to and sign a service contract

- discuss the costs of suggested services

- come up with a plan of care that shows the person's diagnosis (what is wrong), functional limitations (what the person can and cannot do), medications, diet, what services are provided by agency, advice about care, and list of equipment needed

- give you a written copy of the plan of care

- send a copy of the plan of care to the person's doctor

- select and send the right caregivers, only to the level of care needed, to the person's home

- adjust services to meet changing needs

Expect the Agency to:

- be an advocate, advisor, and service planner and to share information with you

- give a full professional assessment

- be in touch with the care receiver's doctor as part of the assessment process

- have knowledge of long-term-care services and how to pay for them

- fill out the necessary paperwork for any funded benefits

- show no bias or favor to service providers who may have contracts with the agency

- provide confidential treatment that will not be talked about with others

- provide a written account of care when you ask for it

- have a proven track record of being honest, reliable, and trusted if the agency handles the person's money

Checklist Things to Do Before Selecting an Agency

✓ Interview several agencies.

✓ Get references and CHECK THEM.

✓ Make a list of services you want and ask the agency how much they will cost.

✓ Ask the agency to explain the steps in the care management process and how long each will take.

✓ Understand how and when you can contact the care manager.

✓ Find out if the agency has a system for sending another aide if the regular one doesn't show up.

✓ Ask if the agency will replace the aide if the person in your care does not get along with the original aide.

✓ Ask about the qualifications of personnel and their ongoing training.

✓ Ask how the quality of services are monitored.

✓ Ask for the services the person in care needs, even if the insurance company is trying to control costs.

✓ Be aware that if a social service agency is providing the care services, they may limit you to the particular services that they provide.

✓ Ask for a disclosure of referral-fee arrangements with nursing homes or other care facilities.

✓ Know the process for lodging complaints against the agency with the state ombudsman or long-term care office at the state level.

✓ Contact the local/state Division for Aging Services to check for complaints against a particular agency.

Hire Someone Privately—A Personal Assistant

Even if you decide not to use an agency, a health care professional can help you decide how to prepare the home. They can give advice about needed supplies and where to purchase them and help set up a care program. However, when you hire someone privately, you must assume payroll responsibility, complete required government forms (such as Social Security), decide on fringe benefits, track travel expenses, and provide a detailed list of tasks to be done.

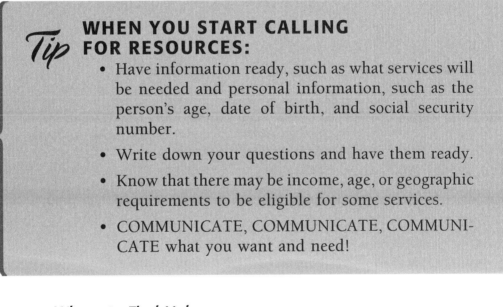

Tip

WHEN YOU START CALLING FOR RESOURCES:

- Have information ready, such as what services will be needed and personal information, such as the person's age, date of birth, and social security number.

- Write down your questions and have them ready.

- Know that there may be income, age, or geographic requirements to be eligible for some services.

- COMMUNICATE, COMMUNICATE, COMMUNICATE what you want and need!

Where to Find Help

- the Yellow Pages under Nurses, Nursing Services, Social Service Organizations, Home Health Services, and Senior Services; the newspaper's personal services column in classified ads

- commercial agencies, which operate like temp agencies, screen applicants and provide you with a list of candidates

- nonprofit agencies, such as the Visiting Nurse Association, which may charge a fee on a sliding scale (based on ability to pay)

- public health nursing through a county social service department (if you have no insurance or money)

- a hospital discharge planner

- hospital-based home health agencies

- the school of nursing at a local community college

- college employment offices

- hospices (call the National Hospice Organization)

- nurses' registries

- Catholic Charities, Jewish Family Services, and other faith-based groups

- the American Red Cross

- churches, synagogues, mosques

- a nearby nursing home employee who seeks part-time work

- an adult relative whom you would pay a fair hourly wage for services

Types of Health Care Professionals

Registered Nurse (RN)—2–4 years of college education and is licensed by the state Board of Nursing Examiners

Licensed Practical Nurse (LPN)—has finished a 1-year course of study and is licensed by the state Board of Licensed Vocational Nurses

Certified Nurses Aide (CNA)—has completed 70 hours of classes and 50 hours of clinical practice in a nursing center setting; must pass a test and register with the State Board of Nursing

Home Health Aide—has training and requirements that are different from state to state; is screened on the basis of work experience

Someone who is taking classes or is in an educational or training program that leads to one of the above professions might be able to help with care.

Tax Rules If You Hire Privately

- If you paid more than $1,400 in 2005 and $1,500 in 2006, you are required to pay Medicare and Social Security tax.

- You may use federal tax Form 1040 to pay the Social Security, Medicare, and Federal Unemployment (FUTA) taxes. Ask the Internal Revenue Service for the *Household Employer's Tax Guide.*

- For tax information, call the Social Security office. Look in the front of your phone book under State Government.

How to Screen a Personal Hire

- Check licenses, training, experience, and references.

- Be sure the person who is applying for the job (the applicant) is insured for malpractice or liability.

- Run a criminal background check and a driving record check (through a private investigator). Also, ask to see the person's insurance card.

- Find out if the person has a special skill (for example, working with people who are paralyzed or have a terminal illness).

- Decide whether the person is someone who can meet the emotional needs of the person in your care.

- Consider his or her personal habits.
- Find out if he or she is a smoker or a nonsmoker.

> **NOTE** You can hire a private investigator to look into public records and check on the person's education and professional licenses, driving history, and previous employers. This service can be obtained anywhere in the country.

Questions to Ask of the Applicant's References:

When you are ready to hire someone, ask for the names of people who can tell you about this person's personal and work habits. Here are some questions you can ask:

- How long have you known the person?
- Did the person work for you?
- Is the person reliable, on time for work, able to adjust to changes, able to be trusted, and polite?
- How does the person handle disagreements and emergencies?
- How well does the person follow instructions, respond to requests, and take advice?

Perform All Caregiving Duties Yourself

If you decide to provide all the caregiving yourself, you can receive training at the following places:

- social service agencies
- hospitals
- community schools
- the American Red Cross

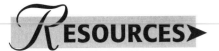

RESOURCES >

Eldercare Locator
(800) 677-1116
www.eldercare.gov
Provides information about local support resources providing services to the elderly.

Family Caregiver Alliance
690 Market Street, Suite 600
San Francisco, CA 94104
(800) 445-8106; (415) 434-3388; Fax: (415) 434-3508
www.caregiver.org
E-mail: info@caregiver.org
Resource center for caregivers of brain-impaired adults. The Web site provides information on services for families of people with brain disorders.

National Family Caregivers Association
10400 Connecticut Avenue, Suite 500
Kensington, MD 20895-3944
(800) 896-3650; (301) 942-6430
www.thefamilycaregiver.org
E-mail: info@thefamilycaregiver.org
The Association supports, empowers, educates, and speaks up for more than 50 million Americans who care for a chronically ill, aged, or disabled person.

Home Care Agencies/Hiring Help

The Center for Applied Gerontology, Council for Jewish Elderly
3003 W. Touhy Avenue
Chicago, IL 60645.
(773) 508-1000
E-mail: cag@cje.net
www.cje.net/professional/cag_orderform_2.pdf
Offers a 32-page pamphlet "Someone Who Cares: A Guide to Hiring an In-Home Caregiver" $9.95 plus $3.50 shipping and handling.

National Association for Home Care
228 Seventh Street, SE
Washington, DC 20003
(202) 547-7424
www.nahc.org
Provides referrals to state associations, which can refer callers to local agencies. Offers publications, including the free pamphlet "How to Choose a Home Care Agency: A Consumer's Guide." Information on finding help, interviewing, reference checking, training, being a good manager, maintaining a good working and personal relationship, problems that might arise and how best to solve them, service dogs, assistive technology, and tax responsibilities. Contains sample forms and letters.

Publications

Avoiding Attendants from Hell: A Practical Guide to Finding, Hiring and Keeping Personal Care Attendants by June Price.

Managing Personal Assistants: A Consumer Guide, published by Paralyzed Veterans of America. To purchase a copy call (888) 860-7244, or download online at www.pva.org/cgi-bin/pvastore/products.cgi?id=2

If you don't have access to the Internet, ask your local library to help you locate a Web site.

Preparing the Home

Preparing the Home

Adapting the home for a person who is partially or fully disabled can be a difficult process or a simple process. In general, the more adaptations (changes) that can be made early on—with a view toward future needs—the easier life will be for everyone concerned. Few caregivers can afford to remodel a home totally. Yet, it is important for readers to be aware of the "ideal" as they plan the changes that make sense for their situations.

Here we present suggestions—from architects who specialize in elder care housing, occupational therapists, and others—for setting up the best home care conditions.

Safety, Safety, Safety

"In 2003, almost 13,000 people 65 and older died from a fall. Of those, 7,500 occurred in the home and 2,500 in a residental setting. . . . Among all age groups 'falls' ranked as the second leading cause of unintentional injury deaths in the United States. Of those who survive a fall, 20–30 percent will suffer debilitating injuries that affect them the rest of their lives" (Source: National Safety Council, Report on Injuries in America, 2003).

The main concern in any home is safety. Accidents can happen but with a little planning can be prevented. Take a close look at the home where you will provide care. You may want to ask a relative or friend to look at it with you to make sure you haven't overlooked any safety hazards.

NOTE ▶ Leave a blanket, pillow, and phone on the floor out of the flow of foot traffic. In case of a fall, the person in your care can stay warm and call for help. In this age of technology, a care receiver who spends time alone should always have a cell phone with him.

As you plan for safety in the home, think about what you will need now and what you will need in the future. For example, furniture that works well for a 65-year-old may need to be changed or replaced later as the person loses strength. Your first concern is to make the home as safe as possible.

As you make changes to the home, don't forget your own comfort and ease. Making life easier for yourself means you will have more time to provide care or to rest. In the long run, this will improve the overall setting for care.

The Home Setting

The ideal home for the care of elderly or disabled persons is on one level (ground floor). Having more than one floor is all right as long as there is an elevator or other approved lift device. The ideal care home is laid out so that the caregiver and the person in care can see each other from other rooms.

Safety

For the safest home, follow as many of these steps as possible:

- Remove any furniture that is not needed.

- Place the remaining furniture so that there is enough space for a walker or wheelchair. This will avoid the need for an elderly or disabled person to move around coffee tables and other barriers. Move any low tables that are in the way.

- Once the person in your care has gotten used to where the furniture is, do not change it.

- Make sure furniture will not move if it is leaned on.

- Make sure the armrests of a favorite chair are long enough to help the person get up and down.

- Add cushioning to sharp corners on furniture, cabinets, and vanities.

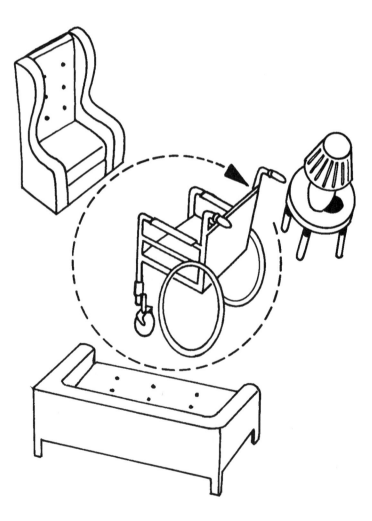

▶ To accommodate a wheelchair, arrange furniture 5^1/$_2$ feet apart.

- Make chair seats 20" high. (Wood blocks or a wooden platform can be placed under large, heavy furniture to raise it to this level.)

- Have a carpenter install railings in places where a person might need extra support. (Using a carpenter can ensure that railings can bear a person's full weight and will not give way.)

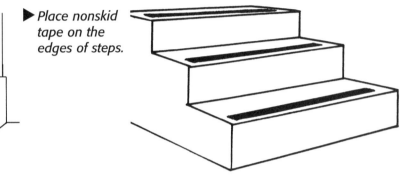

▶ *Place nonskid tape on the edges of steps.*

▲ *Always provide railings along stairways. When possible, extend the handrail past the bottom and top step.*

- Place masking or colored tape on glass doors and picture windows.

- Use automatic night-lights in the rooms used by the person in your care.

- Clear fire-escape routes.

- Provide smoke alarms on every floor and outside every bedroom.

- Place a fire extinguisher in the kitchen.

- Think about using monitors and intercoms.

- Place nonskid tape on the edges of stairs (and consider painting the edge of the first and last step a different color from the floor).

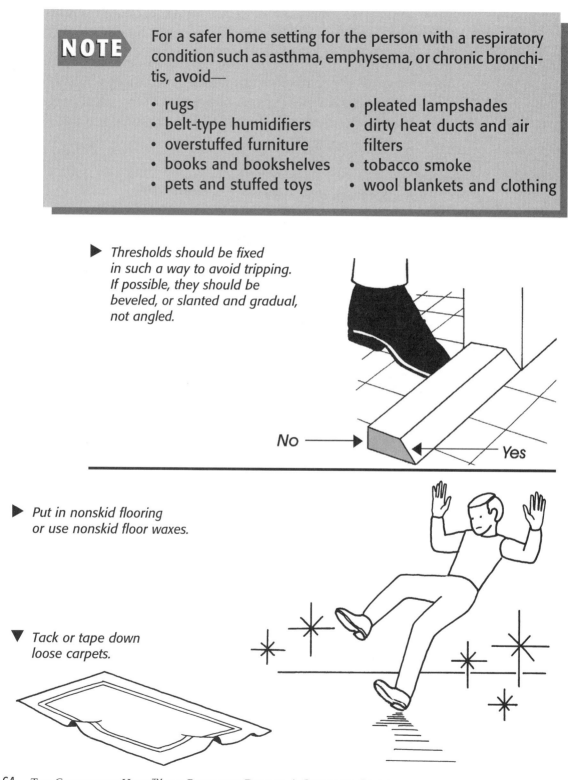

NOTE For a safer home setting for the person with a respiratory condition such as asthma, emphysema, or chronic bronchitis, avoid—

- rugs
- belt-type humidifiers
- overstuffed furniture
- books and bookshelves
- pets and stuffed toys
- pleated lampshades
- dirty heat ducts and air filters
- tobacco smoke
- wool blankets and clothing

▶ *Thresholds should be fixed in such a way to avoid tripping. If possible, they should be beveled, or slanted and gradual, not angled.*

No ⟶   ⟵ Yes

▶ *Put in nonskid flooring or use nonskid floor waxes.*

▼ *Tack or tape down loose carpets.*

- It is easier to walk on thin-pile carpet than on thick pile. Avoid busy patterns.
- Be sure stairs have even surfaces with no metal strips or rubber mats to cause tripping.
- Remove all hazards that might lead to tripping.
- Tape or tack electrical and telephone cords to walls.
- Adjust or remove rapidly closing doors.

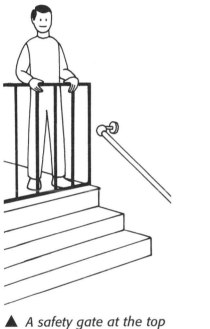

▲ *A safety gate at the top of stairs can prevent falls.*

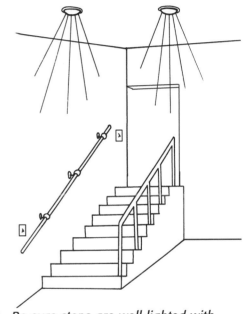

▲ *Be sure steps are well lighted with light switches at both the top and bottom of the stairs.*

- Place protective screens on fireplaces.
- Cover exposed hot-water pipes.
- Provide enough no-glare lighting—indirect is best.
- Place light switches next to room entrances so the lights can be turned on before entering a room. Consider "clap-on" lamps beside the bed.
- Use 100 to 200–watt lightbulbs for close-up activities (but make sure lamps can handle the extra wattage).

 An 85-year-old needs about three times the amount of light a 15-year-old needs to see the same thing. Contrasting colors play a big part in seeing well. As much as possible, the color of furniture, toilet seats, counters, etc., should be different from the floor color.

- Plan for extra outdoor lighting for good nighttime visibility, especially on stairs and walkways.
- If possible, install a carbon monoxide (CO) detector that sounds an alarm when dangerous levels of CO are reached. Call the **American Lung Association**, (800) LUNG USA, for details.
- Work out an emergency escape plan in case of fire.

 If the person in your care is on life support equipment, install a backup electrical power system and have a plan of action in case the power goes out.

Comfort and Convenience

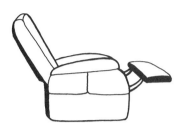

▲ *Think about getting a power-assisted recliner that allows the power-assist feature to be turned off.*

▶ *Install entry ramps. Rails can be added for more safety.*

- For persons who are frail or wheelchair-bound, put in automatic door openers.

- For a person with a wheelchair or a walker, allow at least 18–24″ clearance from the door on landings.

- Plan to leave enough space (a minimum of 32″ clear) for moving a hospital bed and wheelchair through doorways.

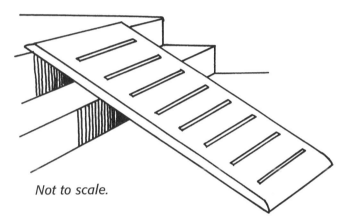

Not to scale.

NOTE ▶ If you are redoing or building a new two-story house, have the contractor frame in the shell of the elevator and then add the elevator unit later when needed. Use the space as a closet for now.

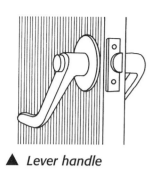

▲ Lever handle

- To widen doorways, remove the molding and replace regular door hinges with offset hinges. Whenever possible, remove doors.

- Put lever-type handles on all doors.

- If a person who is disabled must be moved from one story to another, install a stair elevator.

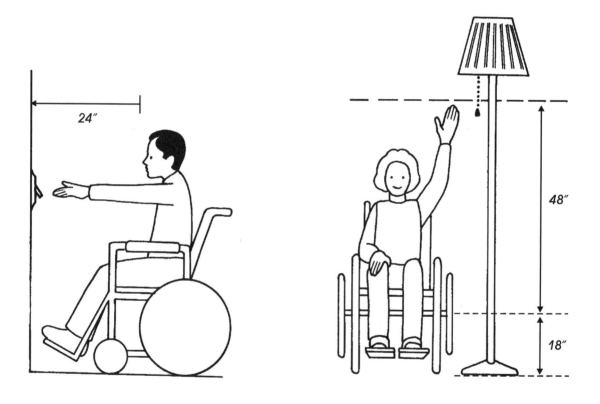

▲ *A person can reach forward about 24" from a seated position. Between 18" and 48" from the floor is the ideal position for light switches, telephones, and mailboxes.*

The Bathroom

Many accidents happen in bathrooms, so check the safety of the bathroom that you will use for home care.

Safety

▶ *Install grab bars beside the toilet, along the edge of the sink, and in the tub and shower according to the needs of each person.*

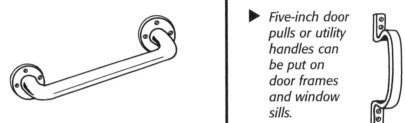

▶ *Five-inch door pulls or utility handles can be put on door frames and window sills.*

- Cover all sharp edges with rubber cushioning.

- Put lights in the medicine cabinets so mistakes are not made when taking medicine.

- Remove locks on bathroom doors.

- Use nonskid safety strips or a nonslip bath mat in the tub or shower.

- Think about putting a grab rail on the edge of the vanity. (Do not use a towel bar.)

- Remove glass shower doors or replace them with un-breakable plastic.

- Use only electrical appliances with a ground fault in-terrupted (GFI) feature.

- Install GFI electrical outlets.

- Set the hot water thermostat below 120° F.

- Use faucets that mix hot and cold water, or paint hot water knobs/faucets red.

- Insulate (cover) hot water pipes to prevent burns.

- Put in toilet guard rails or provide a portable toilet seat with built-in rails. (📖 See *Equipment and Supplies*, p. 86.)

Comfort and Convenience

- If possible, the bathroom should be in a straight path from the bedroom of the person in your care.
- Put in a ceiling heat lamp.
- Place a telephone near the toilet.
- Provide soap-on-a-rope or put a bar of soap in the toe of a nylon stocking and tie it to the grab bar.
- Place toilet paper within easy reach.
- Try to provide enough space for two people at the bathroom sink.
- If possible, have the sink 32″–34″ from the floor.
- Use levers instead of handles on faucets.
- Provide an elevated (raised) toilet seat.

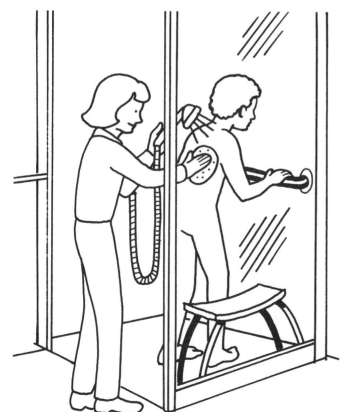

◀ *If possible, have a shower stall that is large enough for two people. Use a hand-held shower head with a very long hose and adjustable jet stream. Put a tub seat or bench in the shower stall.*

The Kitchen

Many of the following suggestions are made to fit the needs of people who are handicapped or elderly who are able to help in the kitchen.

Safety

- Use an electric teakettle.
- Set the water-heater temperature at 120°F.
- Use a single-lever faucet that can balance water temperature.
- Provide an area away from the knife drawer and the stove where the person in your care can help prepare food.
- Use a microwave oven whenever possible (but not if a person with a pacemaker is present).
- Ask the gas company to modify your stove to provide a gas odor that is strong enough to alert you if the pilot light goes out.
- If possible, have the range controls on the front of the stove.
- Provide a step stool, never a chair, to reach high shelves.

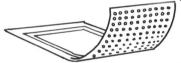

▲ *Cover the floor with a nonslip surface or use a nonskid mat near the sink, where it may be wet.*

Comfort and Convenience

- Use adjustable-height chairs with locking casters.
- Install a Lazy Susan® (swivel plate) in corner cabinets.
- Set up cabinets to reduce bending and reaching.
- Put in a storage wall rather than upper cabinets.
- For easy access, replace drawer knobs with handles.

▶ *Use "reachers"—devices for reaching objects in high or low places without stretching, bending, or standing on a stool.*

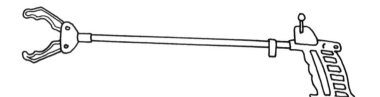

▶ *A cutting board placed over a drawer provides an easy-to-reach surface for a person in a wheelchair.*

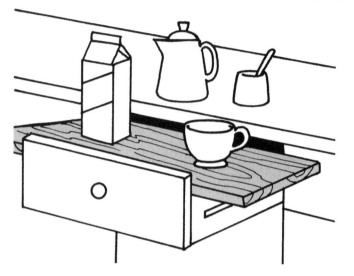

- Place a wire rack on the counter to reduce back strain from reaching dishes.

- Adapt one counter for wheelchair access as pictured above.

- Remove doors under the sink to allow for wheelchair access; also cover exposed pipes.

- Create different counter heights by putting in folding or pull-out surfaces.

- If bending is difficult, consider a wall oven.

- Use suspension systems for heavy drawers.

- Put pullout shelves in cabinets.

- If possible, use a fridge that has the freezer on the bottom.

- Prop the front of the fridge so that the door closes by itself. (If necessary, reverse the way the door swings.)

The Bedroom

Ideally, provide three bedrooms—one for the person in care, one for yourself, and one for the home health aide. Also

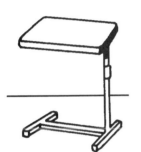

▲ *Provide an adjustable over-the-bed table like the ones used to serve meals in hospital rooms.*

- Put in a monitor to listen to activity in the room of the person in your care. (Most are inexpensive and are portable.)
- Make the bedroom bright and cheerful.
- Make sure enough heat (65° F at night) and fresh air are available.
- Provide a firm mattress.
- Provide TV and radio.
- Think about having a fish tank for fun and relaxation.
- Use throwaway pads to protect furniture.
- Install blinds or shades that darken the room.
- Place closet rods 48″ from the floor.
- Provide a chair for dressing.
- Keep a flashlight at the bedside table.
- Provide a bedside commode with a 4″ foam pad on the seat for comfort.
- Hang a bulletin board with pictures of family and friends where it can be easily seen.
- Provide a sturdy chair or table next to the bed for help getting in and out of bed.

- Make the bed 22″ high and place it securely against a wall. Or use lockable wheels. This will allow the person to get up and down safely.

- Use blocks to raise a bed's height, but be sure to make them steady so they don't move.

▶ *Bedside commode and bed with trapeze bar.*

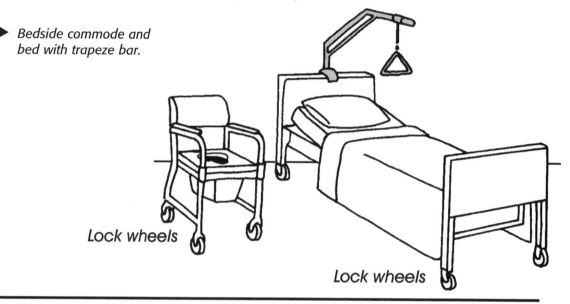

Lock wheels

Lock wheels

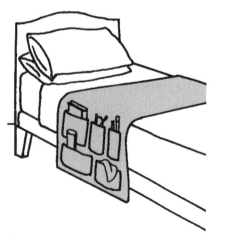

▲ *Make a bed organizer to hold facial tissues, lotion, and other items needed at the bedside. Do this by attaching pockets to a large piece of fabric spread across the bed.*

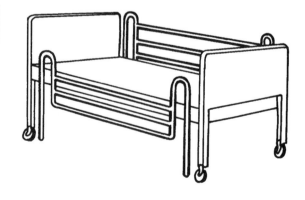

▲ *If all the care is at the bedside, consider a hospital bed. This will be helpful for both you and the person in your care.*

The Telephone

Call your local phone company's special-needs department or visit a store that sells phones and related products. Inquire about

- increasing the size of the numbers on your phone dial so they can be seen and used more easily

▶ *Telephone with enlarged numbers*

- a phone cradle
- step-by-step, large-size instructions for using the phone
- handsets with amplifiers that will make it easier to hear
- signal devices, such as lights that flash when a call is coming in
- TTY (text telephone yoke), a telephone device for the hard of hearing
- a portable phone (to keep out of reach of a person who is confused)
- speed-dial buttons with names or pictures of friends and family instead of numbers
- a one-line phone that automatically connects to a preset number when the button is pressed
- a list of emergency numbers and medicines beside the telephone (📖 See *Setting Up a Plan of Care*, p. 117, for a sample.)

- clear instructions on how to direct emergency personnel to the street address of the house

- a personal emergency response system to signal a friend or emergency service

> **NOTE** Some communities provide a free telephone reassurance service. TRS will make a brief, daily telephone call to persons who are elderly or disabled to reassure them and to share crime prevention information. Call your local police department or the Area Agency on Aging.

Outdoor Areas

Safe outdoor areas are important, especially for those who are frail or elderly and are mobile. Safety features should include the following:

- ramps for access on ground that is not level or even

- a deck with a sturdy railing

- alarmed or locked outside doors

- a key hidden outside

- enough light to see walkway hazards at night

- nonslip step surfaces in good repair

- stair handrails fastened to their fittings

- step edges marked with reflective paint

- a hedge or fence around the yard and dangerous areas like pools or streams

In addition, unplug or remove power tools.

RESOURCES ▸

AARP
601 E Street, NW
Washington, DC 20049
(800) 424-3410
www.aarp.org
Call or write for the booklet, The Do-Able, Renewable Home. *Members can receive one copy at no charge.*

Area Agency on Aging
Your local Area Agency on Aging provides home safety resources.

Center for Universal Design
North Carolina State University
Box 8613
Raleigh, NC 27695-8613
(800) 647-6777; (919) 515-3082 (V/TTY)
Fax: (919) 515-3023
www.design.ncsu.edu\cud
E-mail: cud@ncsu.edu
Established by the National Institute on Disability and Rehabilitation Research (NIDRR) to improve the quality and availability of housing for people with disabilities. Services include information, referral service, training and education, technical design assistance, and publications.

Metropolitan Center for Independent Living, Inc. (MCIL)
1600 University Avenue West, Suite 16
St. Paul, MN 55104-3825
(651) 603-2029
www.wheelchairramp.org
E-mail: jimwi@mcil-mn.org
Web site features How to Build Wheelchair Ramps for Homes, *an online manual for the design and construction of wheelchair ramps.*

National Association of Home Builders Research Center
(800) 638-8556; (301) 249-4000
www.nahbrc.org
Call for its book A Comprehensive Approach to Retrofitting Houses for a Lifetime, *$15 plus postage and handling.*

National Institute for Rehabilitation Engineering
P.O. Box 1088
Hewett, NJ 07421
(800) 736-2216; (973) 853-6585 Fax (928) 832-2894
www.theoffice.net/nire
E-mail: nire@theoffice.net

Paralyzed Veterans of America
801 18th Street NW
Washington, DC 20006-3517
(800) 424-8200
www.pva.org
Not just for veterans, not just for paralysis. Ask for the Architecture Program.

Check with local police to find out if they manage a **Senior Locks Program**. This program can install deadbolt locks and other security devices for homeowners 55 and older who meet federal income guidelines.

Equipment and Supplies

Equipment and Supplies

To provide proper at-home care, you will need to have certain supplies, which fall into two categories:

- *general medical supplies*
- *durable medical equipment*

Before buying anything or signing any contract for rental, talk to the doctor, physical or occupational therapist, or nurse. Salespeople may not be trained to assess what the person in your care may need. Occupational therapists can advise on other low-cost substitutes for expensive equipment. With the proper doctor's orders (referrals) and records, some equipment is covered by Medicare or private insurance. Call your insurance carrier to check if the equipment is covered and follow the company's rules for getting approval before buying.

Where to Buy Needed Supplies

Buy medical equipment and supplies from dealers that are well-established outlets and known for good service. Be sure to get advice about where to buy from your health care professionals or hospital discharge planner. To compare prices, use the chart on page 94 as a sample worksheet.

Look in the Yellow Pages under Surgical Appliances, Physicians and Surgeons, Equipment & Supplies, and First Aid Supplies. Outlets include:

- surgical supply stores
- pharmacies

- hospitals

- home health care agencies

- department stores and large-chain discount stores

- medical supply catalogs

Where to Borrow

For short-term use, think about borrowing equipment from the following local groups:

- Parkinson Disease Support Groups

- Salvation Army

- Red Cross

- Visiting Nurses Association

- home health care agencies

- National Easter Seal Society

- Muscular Dystrophy Association

- American Cancer Society

- charity organizations

- religious organizations, senior centers, leisure clubs

NOTE Never buy equipment from a someone who calls you on the phone to sell something. Do not buy from a door-to-door salesperson. Do not buy from a person who calls even before you know what equipment you will need. Beware of people who contact you unrequested about electric wheelchairs, scooters, etc.

Checklist **General Supplies***

- ✓ antibacterial hand cleaner (kills germs)
- ✓ bacteriostatic ointment (stops the growth of germs)
- ✓ bandages, gauze pads, tape
- ✓ blankets (2 or 3)
- ✓ cotton balls and swabs
- ✓ toothbrush, toothpaste
- ✓ denture or dental care items
- ✓ kidney-shaped basin for oral care
- ✓ container for disposing of syringes (needles)
- ✓ disposable Chux underpad that keeps moisture out, for bed protection
- ✓ draw sheets for use in turning someone in bed
- ✓ finger towels and washcloths
- ✓ foam rubber pillows
- ✓ head pillows
- ✓ heating pad
- ✓ hydrogen peroxide
- ✓ ice bag

- ✓ lotion
- ✓ 4 bed sheets (at least)
- ✓ oral laxative
- ✓ poster with first aid procedures
- ✓ pressure pad and pump
- ✓ sterile disposable gloves
- ✓ rubbing alcohol
- ✓ seat belts (to prevent sliding down in a chair)
- ✓ shower cap
- ✓ soap for dry skin
- ✓ thermometers
- ✓ tissues
- ✓ disposable underpants
- ✓ incontinence briefs
- ✓ panty liners
- ✓ toilet paper tongs to take care of personal hygiene
- ✓ waterproof sheeting
- ✓ roll belt restraint
- ✓ gait/transfer belt
- ✓ Medic Alert® identification

*As needed.

How to Pay

Be creative in seeking help to pay for equipment.

- Ask the doctor to write an order for a home health evaluation (assessment), including what equipment may be needed.
- Find out if the equipment is partly or completely covered by private health insurance with home care benefits.
- Check state retirement and union programs.

 Medicare rules are subject to change.

Medicare does not help pay for assistive devices, but does pay for durable medical equipment in some cases. To be covered, the equipment must be prescribed by a doctor and it must be medically necessary. It must be useful only to the sick or injured person and must be reusable. Medicare will pay for the rental of certain items for no more than 15 months. After that time, you may buy the equipment from the supplier. If the person in your care has met the deductible, Medicare will pay 80% of the approved charges on the rental, purchase, and service of equipment that the doctor has ordered.

 GETTING ORGANIZED

Keep supplies together that are used often and keep a list of supplies so you can easily replace them.

 Be ready for emergencies. Have on hand a flashlight, a battery-run radio, a battery-run clock, fresh batteries, extra blankets, candles with holders, matches, a manual can opener, and bottled water.

Medical Equipment

You will need to provide special equipment for different rooms in the house, as well as equipment to increase the person's ability to get around.

Equipment for the Bedroom

The equipment you need depends on the person's medical condition. This equipment might include some of the items listed below.

- **hospital bed**—allows positioning (adjusting) that is not possible in a regular bed and aids in resting and breathing more comfortably and getting in and out of bed more easily

- **alternating pressure mattress**—reduces pressure on skin tissue

- **egg crate or memory foam mattress topper**—reduces pressure and improves air circulation

- **portable commode chair**—for ease of toileting at the bedside

- **trapeze bar**—provides support and a secure hand-hold while changing positions

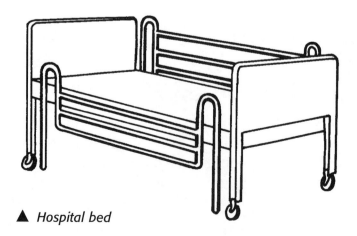

▲ *Hospital bed*

- **transfer board**—a smooth board for independent or assisted transfer from bed to wheelchair, toilet, or portable commode

- **hydraulic lift**—for use on a person who is difficult to move

- **over-the-bed table**—provides a surface for eating, reading, writing, and game playing (could be an adjustable ironing board)

- **mechanical or electric lift chair**—for help getting up from a chair

- **blanket support**—a wire support that keeps heavy bed linens off injured areas or the feet

- **urinal and bed pan**—for toileting in the bed

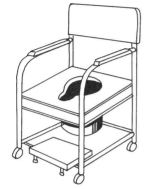

▲ *Portable commode chair*

A sturdy cardboard box placed under the covers keeps the feet and lower legs free of sheets while the person is being turned. Or you can buy the item from a dealer.

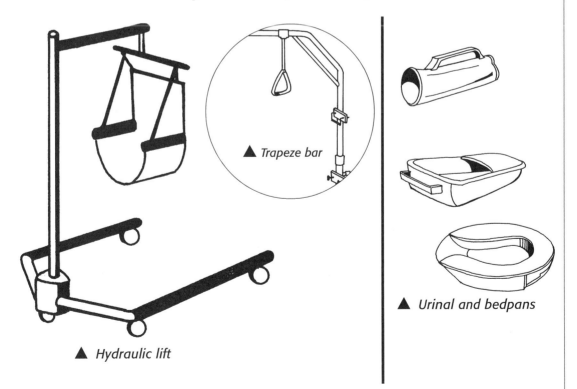

▲ *Trapeze bar*

▲ *Hydraulic lift*

▲ *Urinal and bedpans*

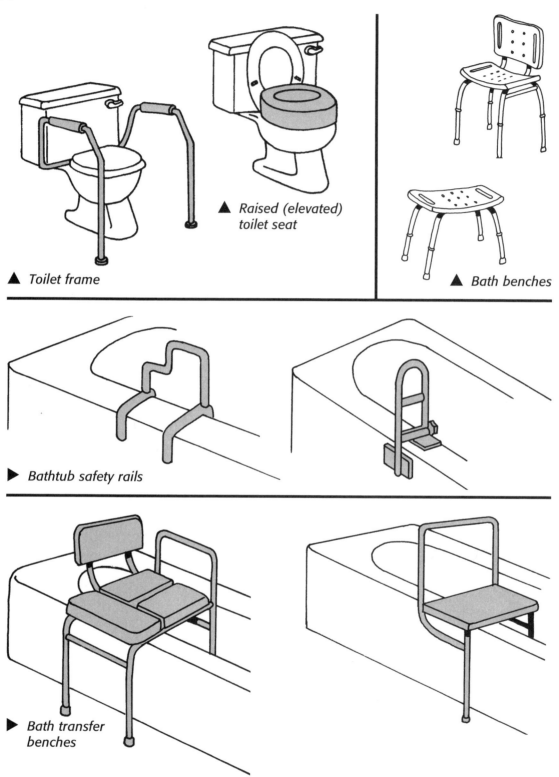

▲ Raised (elevated) toilet seat

▲ Toilet frame

▲ Bath benches

▶ Bathtub safety rails

▶ Bath transfer benches

Equipment for the Bathroom

The equipment you will need depends on the person's needs. You should consider providing the following:

- **raised (elevated) toilet seat**—a seat used to assist a person who has difficulty getting up or down on a toilet (available in molded plastic and clamp-on models for different toilet bowl styles)

- **commode aid**—a device that acts as an elevated toilet seat when used with a splash guard, or as a commode when used with a pail

- **toilet frame**—a freestanding unit that fits over the toilet and provides supports on either side for ease in getting up and down

- **grab bars for tub and shower**—properly installed wall-mounted safety bars that hold a person's weight

- **safety mat and strips**—rough vinyl strips that stick to the bottom of the tub and shower to prevent slipping

- **hand-held shower hose**—a movable shower hose and head that directs the flow of water to all parts of the body

- **bath bench**—aid for a person who has difficulty sitting down in or getting up from the bottom of the tub

- **bath transfer bench**—a bench that goes across the side of the tub and allows a person to get out of the tub easily

- **bathtub safety rails**—support for getting in and out of the tub

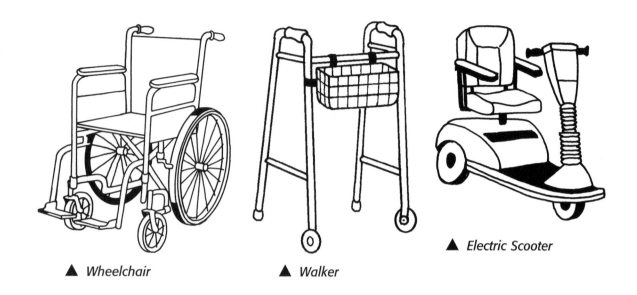

▲ Wheelchair   ▲ Walker   ▲ Electric Scooter

Mobility Aids

Mobility aids include devices that help a person move around without help. They also help the caregiver transfer the person in and out of bed and from bed to a chair.

They include

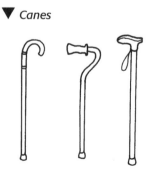

▼ Canes

- a wheelchair with padding and removable arms

- a walker to help the person keep his or her balance and provide some support

- a 3- or 4-wheel electric scooter

- crutches for use when weight cannot be put on one leg or foot

- a cane to provide light weight-bearing support

- a transfer board (9″ x 24″) for moving someone in and out of bed

- a gait/transfer belt (📖 see how to use on p. 237)

See a physical therapist before buying a cane, walker, or wheelchair. Avoid tripod or quad canes (3- or 4-

point bases). People with PD have trouble using these because canes are too close to the feet or all points don't touch the floor at the same time.

To adjust a cane to the proper height:

- Stand straight with arms hanging at sides.

- Caregiver places cane or walker next to person's arm.

- Top of cane or walker should be as high as the bend in the person's wrist.

Tip

Think about using hiking sticks while walking

- Four-post walkers are not recommended for people with PD. Picking up a walker can cause a backward loss of balance.

- Four-wheeled walkers offer better stability and easier turns. Special features such as large wheels, swivel casters, and hand brakes provide the most stability.

- Walkers with built-in seats and baskets are especially helpful.

Tip

MOBILITY

A baby stroller helps a person maintain balance and provides some support. It is easy to move from room to room, and provides a large surface for carrying items.

Wheelchair Requirements

- safety
- durability
- ease of repair
- attractive appearance

- comfort
- ease of handling
- cushions

> **Tip**
>
> **USING CANES**
> Put Velcro® on the top of a cane and put another piece on counters and bedside tables to keep the cane from falling when not in use.

Wheelchair Attachments

- a brake extension
- elevated leg rests and removable footrests
- armrests that can be taken off

NOTE Some states have enacted lemon laws that cover wheel-chairs and other assistive devices. If you think there is something wrong with the equipment you have bought and you want to find out if it qualifies as a lemon, contact the Attorney General's office in your state to find out about getting a replacement or a refund.

Assistive Devices

For those with poor sight and hearing and other limitations, there are many aids to make life easier. Look into all the options and you will find that your job as caregiver becomes easier too.

Sight Aids

- prism glasses
- magnifying glasses
- prescription glasses

- Braille books and signs
- cassette players and books on tape
- telesensory devices that change printed letters into symbols that can be touched

Listening Aids

- hearing aids (order from an audiologist, or hearing specialist, who allows a free 30-day trial and is a registered dealer)
- sound systems that amplify (make louder)
- telephone amplifiers (for increased volume)
- devices for getting close-captioned TV programs

HELP FOR SPECIAL EQUIPMENT
Investigate whether Medicaid or the Lion's Club in your state can pay for hearing aids.

Eating Aids

- spoons that swivel, for those who have trouble with wrist movement
- foam that can be fit over utensils to increase the gripping surface so that utensils can be lifted more easily
- plate guards or dishes with high sides that make it easier to scoop food onto a spoon
- rocker knives that can cut food with a rocking motion
- food-warming dishes for slow eaters
- mugs with two handles, a cover, a spout, and a suction base

- nosey cups (which are cut down on one side and make it easier to drink without tipping the head back

- spill-proof cups (won't leak if tilted too much or get knocked over)

- nonslip surfaces such as Dycem® (keeps plate from sliding around)

▼ *Eating aids—mug, utensils with built-up handles, food guard, one-hand knife, swivel spoon.*

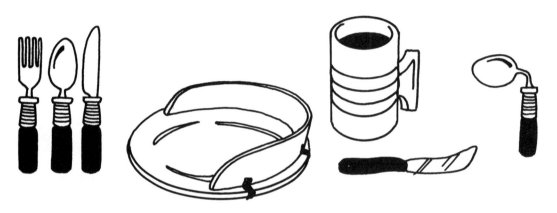

Dressing Aids

- buttonhooks that make buttoning clothes easy

- dressing sticks that make it possible to dress without bending

- long-handled shoe horns so the person doesn't have to bend over when putting on shoes

- sock aids that keep stockings open while they are being put on

(📖 See examples that follow.)

Tip Socks with half tops are easier to put on than mid-calf socks.

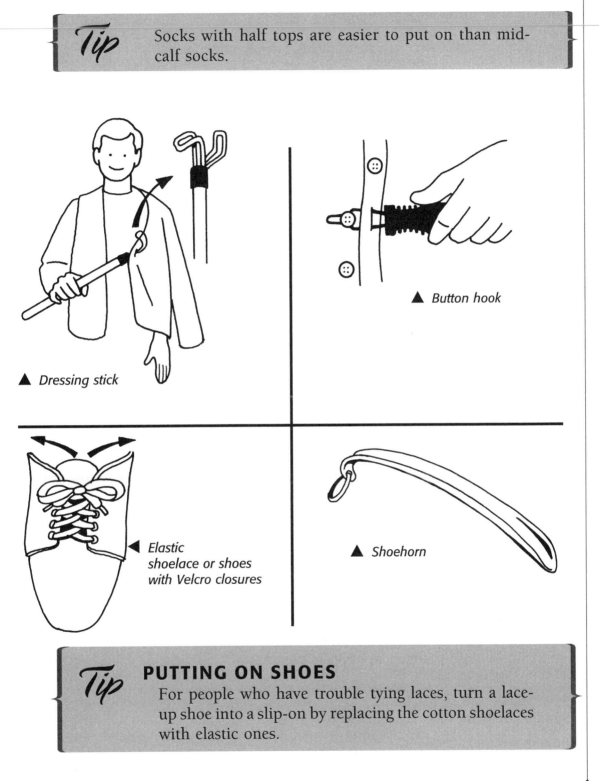

▲ Dressing stick

▲ Button hook

◀ Elastic shoelace or shoes with Velcro closures

▲ Shoehorn

Tip **PUTTING ON SHOES**

For people who have trouble tying laces, turn a lace-up shoe into a slip-on by replacing the cotton shoelaces with elastic ones.

93

Devices for Summoning Help

- touch-tone phones with speed dials
- wireless devices that transmit (send) signals for emergency response
- medical security response systems
- beepers for the caregiver

Homemade Aids and Gadgets

- wrist straps for canes—tape tied on a cane so it can be hung from the wrist while walking upstairs
- kitchen chair trolleys—made by putting casters on a chair and used to move things around easily
- bicycle baskets—strapped to a walker to store necessities and leave the hands free
- an egg carton—to organize pills
- rubber safety mats—ideal for the tub, shower, or any slippery surface; also useful to place on trays and tables for nonslip surface
- key enlargements—put the end of the key that you hold into a large cork for ease of grip
- foot-operated door levers—made by attaching rope to a "stirrup" and tying it to the lever handle
- enlarged handles—handlebar-style grips made with a garden hose, bendable aluminum tubing, a paint-roller cover, or (on small surfaces) a foam hair-curler roller
- language tags—cardboard tags with words that can be used to express needs
- light-switch enlargements—made by putting a rubber pen cap over a light switch
- enlarged pull switches—made by putting a plastic ball over small switches

- clips for canes—spring clips or Velcro® placed on favorite chairs to keep a cane from falling

- bedside rails—wooden rails attached to the floor at right angles on swivel hinges

- pull rope—rope attached to the footboard of the bed to help someone change positions in bed

Specialized Hospital-Type Equipment

- **oxygen tanks**, for use when oxygen is needed as a medication

- **breathing tube (transtracheal oxygen therapy equipment)**, for use when oxygen is delivered into the lungs through a flexible tube that goes from the neck directly into the trachea (sometimes called the windpipe)

- **compressors and hand-held nebulizers (inhalers)**, which reduce medication to a form that can be inhaled

- **suction catheters**, which clear mucus and secretions from the back of the throat when someone cannot swallow

- **home infusion equipment**, or intravenous (IV) therapy, which delivers antibiotics, blood products, chemotherapy, hydration (fluids), pain management, parenteral (IV) nutrition, and specialty medications

Equipment Cost-Comparison Chart *(Example)*

Item	Purchase Price	Rental Fee × Months Needed	Covered by Medicare Yes/No	Vendor
bath stool	$			
bedpan				
bed safety accessories				
cane				
commode				
crutches				
hospital bed				
mattress				
oxygen				
raised toilet seat				
special equipment				
trapeze				
walker				
wheelchair				
3- or 4-wheel scooter				
other				
Totals	$			

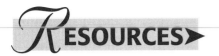

*R*ESOURCES➤

AbilityHub
www.abilityhub.com
Assistive technology for people who have difficulty operating a computer.

ABLEDATA
8630 Fenton Street, Suite 930
Silver Spring, MD 20910-3319
(800) 227-0216; (301) 608-8998; Fax: (301) 608-8958
www.abledata.com
Stores information on thousands of assistive devices for home health care, from eating utensils to wheelchairs. Provides prices, names, and addresses of suppliers.

Adaptive Environments Center Inc.
374 Congress Street, Suite 301
Boston, MA 02210
(617) 695-1225 (v/tty); Fax (617) 482-8099
www.adaptiveenvironments.org
E-mail: info@adaptiveenvironments.org

Alliance for Technology Access
www.ataccess.org
A network of community-based resource centers, developers, vendors, and associates dedicated to providing information and support services to children and adults with disabilities, and increasing their use of standard, assistive, and information technologies. You can order their book Computer Resources for People with Disabilities *online.*

American Occupational Therapy Association (AOTA)
4720 Montgomery Lane
P.O. Box 31220
Bethesda, MD 20824-1220
(301) 652-2682; Fax (301) 652-7711
www.aota.org
Provides consumer publications.

Apple Computer Accessibility
www.apple.com/accessibility
Committed to helping people with disabilities to access their computers.

AT&T Special Needs Center
(800) 872-3883 (TTY)
Provides free directory assistance (with an application) and operator's help dialing for those who have impaired vision or are disabled.

Briggs
(800) 247-2343

Independent Living Research Utilization at TIRR
2323 S. Shepherd, Suite 1000
Houston, TX 77019
(800) 949-4232; (713) 520-0232
www.ilru.org
E-mail: ilru@ilru.org

Lighthouse International for the Blind
111 E. 59th Street
New York, NY 10022
(800) 829-0500; (212) 821-9200
www.lighthouse.org
Provides free information on eye-related diseases and can refer individuals to resources in the community. Free catalog on low-vision aides.

Lumex
(800) 645-5272

Medic Alert®
(800) 432-5378
Offers critically important medical facts about the emblem wearer's condition to emergency personnel 24 hours a day.

Microsoft Accessibility Technology for Everyone
www.microsoft.com/enable
A Web site of products, training, and free resources to make technology accessible to everyone.

National Rehabilitation Information Center for Independence
4200 Forbes Boulevard, Suite 202
Lanham, MD 20706
(800) 346-2742
www.naric.com
E-mail: naricinfo@heitechservices.com
A database of research information about assistive technology and rehabilitation. One-stop shopping for referrals, information, and equipment sources. Fees for some services.

NCM Aftertherapy Catalog
(800) 235-7054

Radio Shack
Carries a variety of alerting devices in stores nationwide.

Sammons-Preston
Bowling Brook, IL
(800) 323-5547

Sears Home Health Care Catalogue
(800) 326-1750 for customer service
To place an order or find a Sears store near you.

Self-Help for Hard of Hearing People (SHHH)
7910 Woodmont Avenue, Suite 1200
Bethesda, MD 20814
(301) 657-2248; (301) 657-2249 (TTY)
Offers information on coping with hearing loss and on hearing aids.

SpeciaLiving Magazine
www.specialiving.com
Online info and store for accessible housing, special products, such as ramps, bathing systems, urinary devices, lifts.

World Institute on Disability
510 16th Street, Suite 100
Oakland, CA 94612
(510) 763-4100; TTY: (510) 208-9496;
Fax: (510) 763-4109
www.wid.org
E-mail: wid@wid.org

For **medical alarms**, consult the phone book or contact your local hospital's long-term care or senior services division.

Part Two: Day by Day

Setting Up a Plan of Care

Setting Up a Plan of Care

A plan of care is a daily record of the care and treatment a person needs after a hospital stay. The plan helps you and the person in your care with caregiving tasks.

When a person leaves a hospital, the discharge planner provides the caregiver with a copy of the doctor's orders and a brief set of instructions for care. The discharge planner also works with a home health care agency to send a nurse, The nurse will evaluate the patient's needs for equipment, personal care, help with shots or medication, etc. The nurse will also work with the entire health care team (including you as the caregiver, a physical therapist, and other specialists) to develop a detailed plan of care.

The plan of care includes the following information:

- diagnosis (the nature of the disease)
- medications
- functional limitations (what the person can and cannot do)
- a list of equipment needed
- special diet
- detailed care instructions and comments
- services the home health care agency provides

The information is presented in a certain order so that the process of care is repeated over and over until it becomes routine. When the plan is kept up to date, it provides a clear record of events that helps solve problems and avoid them.

With a plan, you don't have to rely on your memory. It also allows another person to take over respite care or take your place entirely without too much trouble.

Some of the things you may have to watch and record are:

- *skin color, warmth, and tone (dryness, firmness, etc.)*
- *pressure areas where bedsores can develop (see Activities of Daily Living, p. 174)*
- *breathing, temperature, pulse, and blood pressure*
- *circulation (dark red or blue spots on the legs or feet)*
- *fingernails and toenails (any unusual conditions)*
- *mobility (ability to move around)*
- *puffiness around the eyes and cheeks, swelling of the hands and ankles*
- *appetite*
- *body posture (relaxed, twisted, or stiff)*
- *bowel and bladder function (unusual changes)*
- *motor fluctuation in response to medication timing (see chapter 2)*

Value the Partnerships with the Care Team

The partnerships you form with the health care team, family members, and friends play a major role in meeting the challenges of Parkinson disease. As a caregiver you should be able to talk openly and easily to health care professionals and to the person in your care.

Try to find language that works—good communication between you and the person with PD is very important.

Take Charge of PD

Ideally, try and take an active role in Parkinson disease. Together with the person you are caring for, learn all about the condition—its causes, symptoms, and treatments. The more you understand, the easier it will be to get through the day-to-day problems.

As caregiver, you are a central part of the health care team ensuring that the person with PD can receive the best treatment possible. Other good sources of information include magazines, books, news articles, Web sites, and local organizations (see p. 253 for list).

What Can Caregivers Do?

Try to find the most informed and skilled doctors and other health professionals in your community, people with a real interest in Parkinson disease.

It is important for a person with Parkinson disease to visit his or her doctor regularly for checkups. Whenever possible, go with the person so that you can discuss with the doctor any symptoms or concerns that you may have (see *Using the Health Care Team Effectively,* p. 23).

Try not to expect too much from the person with PD—recognize what she can and cannot do.

Stay calm. A person with PD will have both "good" and "bad" days. Try to listen and be patient and understanding. Allow the person the time and space to finish the tasks and goals he sets for himself.

The symptoms of PD are often made worse by anxiety, stress, and pressure. Don't pressure the person to speed up and don't try to do the tasks yourself.

Plan ahead. Remember that day-to-day tasks may take longer than they used to.

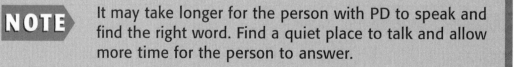

NOTE It may take longer for the person with PD to speak and find the right word. Find a quiet place to talk and allow more time for the person to answer.

Activity Planning

Even if they do *not* have dementia, some people with Parkinson disease may have a lack of interest. They tend to withdraw socially as the disease progresses. Parkinson symptoms that can lead a person to withdraw from normal activities and interaction include—

- freezing (a walking, or gait, problem where feet seem to be "stuck" to the floor)

- frequent falls or fear of falling

- *dysarthria* (low voice volume)

- slowness of thinking

In these cases, it may be useful for the spouse or other primary caregiver to step into the role of "activity director" for the person with PD.

A daily plan can give form and meaning to the person's time and provide an outlet for his or her energy. If possible, the person with PD should personally draw up the plan. If he or she can type or use a computer, writing a plan provides mental and social stimulation and is good exercise of fine-motor skills.

The daily activity plan of Allen—a 74-year-old man who has had Parkinson disease for 14 years—is a sample plan that he says helps him "stay on track."

Morning

1. Get up at 7 a.m.; remember to use the cane to walk to the toilet.

2. Take first daily dose of Parkinson medication with $\frac{1}{2}$ glass water.

3. Get the newspaper, prepare coffee, and eat breakfast.

4. Brush teeth, shave, shower, and dress.

5. Watch morning news show on television.

6. Do stretching and strengthening exercises.

7. Perform household or yard chores.

8. Run errands as scheduled.

9. Take second dose of medication prior to lunch.

Midday and Afternoon

1. Have lunch at nearby cafe.

2. Walk the dog outside for 20 minutes or ride exercise bike.

3. Take a 45-minute nap.

4. Eat a piece of fruit or other snack.

5. Community activity (senior center, volunteer work, support group).

6. Phone a friend or mail a card to someone out-of-town.

7. Take third dose of medication prior to evening meal.

Evening

1. Watch early news and weather on TV.

2. Have dinner at home or with friends.

3. Choose a relaxing activity, such as seeing a movie, playing a computer game, or working a crossword puzzle.

4. Lay out clothes for following day.

5. Take bedtime dose of medications.

6. Listen to relaxing music while preparing for bed.

(See NPF's *Caring and Coping* in **Resources** for more info.)

> **Tip** If wearing-off or freezing episodes happen when you are on an outing, try to sit, relax, and "go with the flow" and wait until it passes.

Recording the Plan of Care

Use a loose-leaf notebook to record the plan of care. Put the doctor's instructions on the inside front cover (always keep the originals). Include in the notebook the types of forms that appear in the following pages of this chapter. These pages should be three-hole punched.

After using your plan of care for one week, make changes as needed and continue to do so as the person's needs change. Always do what works for you and the person in your care. Use notes, pictures, or anything else to describe your responsibilities. Also, use black ink, not pencil, to keep a permanent record.

Daily Activities Record (Sample Form)   Day/Date: _____

Morning _____

_____

Afternoon _____

_____

Naps: Time _____ Place _____

Evening _____

_____

Activities	Yes	No	Where/How/When
Walk	☐	☐	_____
TV	☐	☐	_____
Reading Aloud	☐	☐	_____
Visitors	☐	☐	_____
Calls to Friends/Relatives	☐	☐	_____

Other _____

_____

Bedtime Routine	Yes	No	Where/How
Incontinence Pad/Brief	☐	☐	_____
Medication	☐	☐	_____
Special Pillow/Blanket	☐	☐	_____
Music/Radio/TV	☐	☐	_____
Nightlight	☐	☐	_____
Restraints, Calming Techniques	☐	☐	_____
Urinal/Bedpan	☐	☐	_____
Gates at Doors/on Stairs	☐	☐	_____
Oral/Denture Care	☐	☐	_____
Foot Care	☐	☐	_____

Braces ☐   Fungus ☐   Massage ☐   Ingrown Nails ☐   Nail Care ☐

Meals

Help Needed with Meals _____

Meal Times _____

Special Diet _____

Foods to Avoid _____

Special Utensils _____

Snacks _____

Favorite Foods _____

Location of Meals _____

Daily Care Record (Sample Form)   Day/Date: _____

Daily Activities/Limitations:
Walks Alone _____ Stands Alone _____
Bed Position _____
Equipment Used: Walker ❐   Cane ❐   Wheelchair ❐   Brace ❐
How long _____
ROM/Exercises: Upper Body ❐   Lower Body ❐   Goes Outside ❐

Meals: Special Diet   ❐
Breakfast _____
Lunch _____
Dinner _____
Snack _____
Fluids _____

Treatments
Catheter _____
Oxygen _____
Equipment _____
Physical Therapy _____
Special Precautions _____
Resuscitate ❐   Do Not Resuscitate ❐

Personal Care
Bath: ❐ Bed   ❐ Chair
Shower: ❐ Tub   ❐ Bench
Care of Genitals: _____
Nail Care: ❐ Toes   ❐ Fingers
Oral Care: ❐ Brush Teeth   ❐ Floss Teeth   ❐ Dentures
Hair Care: ❐ Shave   ❐ Bed Shampoo   ❐ Bath/Shampoo
Skin Care: ❐ Lotion Upper Body ❐ Lotion Lower Body ❐ Powdered
Massage: ❐ Head and Shoulder ❐ Leg and Foot   ❐ Back
Bowel Movements _____ Voiding _____ Quantity _____
Temperature _____ Blood Pressure _____ Respiration _____

Comments/Attitudes/Conditions _____
_____
_____

Visitors _____
_____

Activities Schedule for Backup Caregiver (Sample Form)

Personal Needs	Yes	No	Where to Find
Cane	❐	❐	_____
Dentures	❐	❐	_____
Glasses	❐	❐	_____
Hearing aid	❐	❐	_____
Walker	❐	❐	_____

Morning Routine
Breakfast _____ Where Eaten _____
Amount of Help Needed _____
Special Utensils Needed _____
Medications with Meals ❐ _____ Nap ❐ _____
Snack Foods _____ Time of Snack _____

Evening Routine
Dinner _____ Where Eaten _____
Evening Snack _____

Bedtime Routine
Help Needed Undressing ❐ _____ Shower or Bath Needed ❐ _____
Where Clothes Are Stored _____
Where Dentures Are Stored _____
Special Items Needed: _____
Incontinent Pad/Brief ❐ _____ Urinal ❐ _____ Restraints ❐ _____
Special Pillows ❐ _____ Music ❐ _____ Nightlight ❐ _____
Calming Techniques _____

Special Concerns or Equipment
Catheter ❐ _____ Oxygen ❐ _____
Special Precautions _____
Other _____
Resuscitate ❐   Do Not Resuscitate ❐

Be on the Alert for:
Gates on Stairs/Locks on Doors _____
Alarms _____
Other _____
Don't be surprised if: _____

Recording and Managing Medications

Medication management is the most important part of controlling Parkinson symptoms. Knowing what to expect from these medications can be extremely helpful.

- Always be sure that the person in your care takes the medication exactly as prescribed. Keep an accurate list of these medications and when they should be taken. ( See EPDA's *Working Together* in **Resources** for how to keep an accurate record of medications.)

- Never make any changes to these medications without talking to the doctor or specialist first. However, because everyone's treatment needs are different, the specialist may want to try changing the amount or timing of drugs, within certain limits. If you are worried or have any questions, don't be afraid to ask your doctor or pharmacist for advice.

- It is helpful if the person with PD keeps a record of his or her treatment, including whether the medications are effective and have any side effects. Provide help in keeping this diary and add your own observations.

- Learn to recognize changes in symptoms that may, for example, indicate that the person is experiencing wearing-off of their medication.

NOTE Sometimes people with PD take extra levodopa doses to avoid feeling extreme immobility (frozen) due to the wearing-off phenomenon. If you think the person in your care is taking too much medication, mention it to the neurologist for advice on readjusting the dosage.

You must have a careful system for keeping track of medications:

- when medications *should* be given
- *how* they should be given
- when they were *actually* given

The following sample of a weekly medication schedule is a good model to follow. Be sure to fill in the times when (A.M. and P.M.) medications actually were given, and have each caregiver initial them.

Weekly Medication Schedule (Sample Form)

Medication	Date/Time/Initials						
Name, dose, frequency, with or without food	Sat.	Sun.	Mon.	Tues.	Wed.	Thurs.	Fri.
Example							
Stalevo 150mg* *3x daily* • *8 a.m.* • *Noon* • *4 p.m.*							
Sinemet CR 50/200* *1x daily* • *bedtime*							
Stool softener capsule *1x daily* • *8 a.m.*							
Vitamin/mineral capsule *1x daily, with food* • *Noon*							
Artificial tears *2x daily* • *8 a.m.* • *bedtime*							

*These medications contain levodopa and are best absorbed on an empty stomach with $1/2$ cup water. May also be taken with a non-protein snack (cookie, cracker, small fruit serving) if this medication causes nausea (occurs in only 10% of clients).

As you finish your own schedule, be sure to record information from the label of each prescription, including

- days of the week when each medicine must be taken

- number of times per day

- time of day

- whether the medicine is to be taken with or without food

- how much water should be taken with the medicine

Also make a note to yourself about any warnings (for example, "Don't take this medicine with alcohol") and possible side effects (dizziness, confusion, headache, etc.).

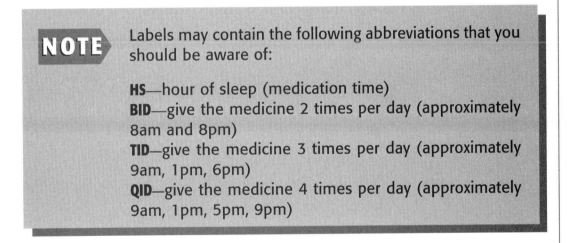

NOTE Labels may contain the following abbreviations that you should be aware of:

HS—hour of sleep (medication time)
BID—give the medicine 2 times per day (approximately 8am and 8pm)
TID—give the medicine 3 times per day (approximately 9am, 1pm, 6pm)
QID—give the medicine 4 times per day (approximately 9am, 1pm, 5pm, 9pm)

Other Cautions

- Never crush drugs without talking to the doctor or pharmacist first. If the person in your care has trouble swallowing medication, ask the doctor if there is another way it can be taken. (See *Using the Health Care Team Effectively*, p. 32.)

- If the person in your care will take the medicine without your help, ask the pharmacist to use easy-open caps on prescription bottles.

- Do not store medicine that will be taken internally (swallowed) in the same cabinet with medicine that will be used externally (lotions, salves, creams, etc.)

- Keep a magnifying glass near the medicine cabinet for reading small print.

- Store most medicine in a cool, dry place—usually not the bathroom.

- Remove the cotton from each bottle so that moisture is not drawn in.

- All medicine more than 12 months' out of date should be flushed down the toilet.

- If childproof containers are too hard to open, ask the pharmacist for containers that are not childproof.

EMERGENCY PREPAREDNESS

Let the local fire station and ambulance company know that a person with disabilities lives at your address. They will have the information on hand and can respond quickly.

Emergency Information

Have this information posted near telephones or on the refrigerator, where it can be used by anyone in the household in case of emergency.

Personal Information

Name _____ Date of Birth _____

Address _____

Phone _____

SS # _____ Supplemental Insurance # _____

Medicaid # _____ Medicare # _____

Current Medications: _____

_____

Exact Location of Do Not Resuscitate Order: _____

Emergency Numbers

Fire _____ Police _____

Ambulance _____ Hospital _____

Doctor _____

Drugstore _____ Open Till _____ Delivers _____

Family Caregiver Work Number _____

Alternate Caregiver _____

Home Health Care Agency _____

Medicare Toll Free Number _____

Insurance _____

Medical Equipment Company _____

Poison Control _____

Friend _____

_____

Neighbor _____ Relative _____

Clergy/Rabbi _____

Transport Number _____ Meals-on-Wheels _____

Shopping Assistance _____

_____

Directions for Driving to the House _____

_____

_____

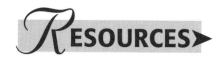

RESOURCES

For more information on the material presented in this chapter, and free brochures on all topics related to Parkinson disease, contact:

American Parkinson Disease Association (APDA)
(800) 223-2732
www.apdaparkinson.org

European Parkinson's Disease Association (EPDA)
www.epda.eu.com

National Parkinson Foundation (NPF)
(800) 327-4545
www.parkinson.org

Caring and Coping is available from the National Parkinson Foundation.

Working Together is available from European Parkinson's Disease Association.

Also see p. 263 for more Web sites that offer education and support.

How to Avoid Caregiver Burnout

How to Avoid Caregiver Burnout

urnout is the complete draining of physical, spiritual, and emotional reserves. It occurs when a caregiver goes beyond exhaustion or depression. Every day, caregivers must remove themselves emotionally from their tasks. Otherwise they risk getting so deeply involved that they burn out. Anyone who cares for a person whose health is getting worse needs understanding, support, and help—from friends, family, and a support group.

*Life doesn't stop after a diagnosis of Parkinson disease—it simply changes and certain adjustments are required. Trust that you may be stronger than you think. Still, as primary caregiver, your most important duty is to save your strength and restore your resources. Remember, you are the one who is going to make it all happen over the long term, so guard your health! (📖 See **Resources for APDA's**, The Fine Art of "Re-creation and Socialization" with Parkinson's Disease.)*

Emotional Burdens You Face

You may think that certain problems were unique to your situation, but they are not. You may resent the loss of your privacy or feel you have no control over the situation. Your caring and concern for the person with Parkinson disease may give you great satisfaction, but every caregiver deals with certain emotional burdens:

- the need to hide grief
- fear of the future
- worry about finances
- lessened ability to solve problems

> **NOTE** Men who undertake caregiving face special problems because often they are not familiar with everyday home-making chores. Additionally, they lose the emotional support of the spouse who is ill and must now be her support. It is especially important for men to seek out support groups.

The Caregiver's Role

As a caregiver, how you can best provide understanding, emotional support, and physical help will depend on what you and the person for whom you are caring decide on together.

If possible, try to agree on the role you will play with the person you care for. The person with Parkinson disease will make the decisions, but you need to be there to offer physical and emotional support when it is called for.

Be prepared for possible changes in Parkinson disease in the future. Your role will probably change as PD progresses.

> **Tip** Whether playing it or simply listening to it, music is good for you. Just like a game of golf or a swim, singing releases endorphins into the bloodstream, making you feel positive. So if in need of stress relief, sing in the shower, sing in the car, sing in a church choir—just sing!

Taking Care of Yourself

As hard as you are working to care for someone else, it is important to remember that you have needs too.

Caregiving can be physically and emotionally draining. It is all too easy to put your own needs at the bottom of the priority list. Make sure you allow yourself some respite. You will find it harder to act in the best interests of the person in your care if you are always tired or depressed.

Allow Time for You

- You cannot do everything, nor should you expect yourself to. Know what you can and can't do and set priorities. Allow yourself some leisure time to rest, relax, and be yourself

- Don't hesitate to turn to family members and friends for emotional support, company, or occasional care-giving support.

- The person with PD should continue with the activities he or she enjoys, and so should you. Try to keep up your hobbies, clubs, activities, and friendships

- Though you have to make some changes in your life, you should not put you life on hold.

- You will have more energy and enthusiasm for your daily routine if your days still include some of the activities you enjoy doing.

Stay Healthy

It is just as important that you look after your own health. Avoid getting run-down. Mild exercise, even just taking a walk, helps your body relax. Add exercising and going out at least once a week to your checklist of things to do.

- It may help to exercise with the person in your care, to make your time together more enjoyable.

- Try to get enough sleep every night. Too little sleep will make you feel run-down and unable to cope with the stress in your life.

- Caregivers can become depressed too. In addition to sadness, fearfulness, and feelings of hopelessness, other signs of depression may include lack of interest in regular activities, inability to sleep, lack of energy, difficulty thinking clearly, and changes in appetite and weight.

- If you are feeling overwhelmed or in need of assistance, speak out. A counselor or medical professional may be able to help

Take a Break

Get help early, not as a last resort. Look into counseling, respite care, or adult day care one or two days a week. Don't be in denial that you need help. Remember to forgive yourself for not being perfect. Understand your grief and seek out someone who understands it.

- When people offer to help, accept the offer. Suggest specific things they can do, such as housecleaning, running errands, or meal preparation.

- Make use of respite care. A wide range of help may be available that can be provided in the home, an adult day care center, or in an extended care facility. Ask your doctor or hospital social worker what kinds of respite care are available in your area.

- Look into whether there are any local support groups where the person with PD can socialize with peers, giving you a well-deserved break. Many PD support groups have regular caregivers-only discussion sessions.

Take a Vacation

If you think you need a vacation, you probably do.

First of all, we should point out the occasional treat and wisdom of traveling *without* the person in your care!

Even if you set aside a few minutes for yourself every day and take a half or full day each week to do things away from your care receiver, there's just nothing that renews your energy and recharges your soul like getting out of town for a few days! Take a cell phone with you, but make it clear that it is for emergencies only, not routine "Where do you keep the cereal?" inquiries. *Do not call home to check in. You are on holiday!*

This is a habit worth building into your care recipient's expectations early in the course of the disease. He will learn that others can help meet needs, whether a family member, friend, or the staff in an assisted living facility. If finances won't permit glamorous travel, just checking into a hotel in a nearby city for a long weekend, dining out, and reading by the pool, can be just the ticket to recharge your caregiving batteries!

Whether a day trip or a longer holiday, if you are going to travel with the person in your care, careful planning can make all the difference in a safe and fun excursion or the kind of trip that makes you wish you'd stayed home. For instance, even if the person in your care walks at home with only the use of a single point cane, it is still wise to reserve a wheelchair when you make air reservations to navigate busy airport corridors and long lines at security check points.

Tip

Many airports no longer have bellmen at luggage claim carousels. *Smarte Carte* luggage strollers are readily available, and can serve dual function as a walker for the person with PD.

Orbitz (www.orbitz.com) is an excellent Web site to compare air, hotel, and rental car prices and features for traveling with someone with a disability. But rather than book on a travel Web site such as Orbitz, Expedia, or Travelocity, it is preferable to book directly with the airline and hotel chain you decide to use. This will ensure that the wheelchair is reserved, etc., and in the case of hotels, offers more lenient cancellation policies if plans change at the last minute. Take advantage of senior discounts or Automobile Association (AAA, CAA) member discounts.

- Pack all meds and an ID card stating that the person you are with has PD in your carry-on bag. (These are available from APDA and NPF.) Carry-on luggage should also contain health insurance cards, doctors' names and phone numbers, and a collapsible cup for water so pills can be easily taken when needed. Some airlines and cruise lines require an authorization letter from a physician stating that persons with significant disability are fit to travel.

- Carry a supply of snacks and a carton of drinks for the person to have when taking medication.

- If you take a long trip, the person with PD should rest on the day before leaving and the day after arriving. It will also help if the person drinks plenty of fluids on the days before and after traveling. This will allow the person to drink less on the day of travel and reduce the number of visits to the bathroom.

- If traveling for a longer period, ask the primary doctor for the name of a neurologist in the place you are going to visit. If there is a time change at your destination, medications should be taken as prescribed, with the same number of hours between doses.

- If traveling abroad, check the person's medical insurance to ensure that there is coverage in the event medical treatment is needed.

> **NOTE** Take more carbidopa/levodopa than the care receiver uses at home on his usual schedule and routine. Extra doses may be required to handle the demands of being away.

- Pace the itinerary so the person with PD does not get overtired and immobile. It is a good idea to plan no more than one or two special events each day. Don't start the days too early. Allow extra time for dressing, eating, and walking in unfamiliar settings.

- Cruises are often ideal vacations for someone with PD. The schedule is leisurely, handicapped cabins are available, and it avoids multiple hotel changes common to other tour groups. There are many onboard activities the person with Parkinson disease can enjoy without your supervision. Some regional Parkinson organizations and support groups sponsor cruise groups for Parkinson patients and their caregivers.

- For American citizens traveling abroad, it helps to know how to contact *American Citizen Services (ACS)* in the offices of U.S. embassies and consulates. They can help with referrals to local doctors, dentists, and hospitals, and guide you through the maze of regulations if there is a death or medical emergency while visiting their country.

- Consider travel adventures closer to home. Exotic foreign destinations often come with numerous challenges for persons with gait and balance problems. Choose flights no longer than 3 hours. Allow a full day each way just for getting there and getting home. Car travel is the most flexible of all vacations, allowing you to choose your own schedule, daily agenda, and bathroom and snack breaks to meet the needs of your person with PD. Hopefully, you've already obtained a handicapped parking permit for easy access when traveling.

Tip

- Take advantage of early boarding privileges, where available. Check in early and request an aisle seat close to the toilet if mobility is a problem.

- Do not hesitate to request a wheelchair or electric cart to get to and from the plane. This will help cut down on the overall fatigue of air travel.

- Carry all the medication that will be needed for the entire trip in your hand luggage. Loss of baggage or flight delays could leave you without enough medication.

Express Your Emotions

As Parkinson disease progresses, one of the toughest challenges for everyone involved will be coping with emotions.

- If you are able, try to talk through problems and don't be afraid to express your feelings. Be honest with yourself and the person with Parkinson disease. Open and frank talks will create a healthier relationship between you.

- You may find it helpful to talk about ways you can help relieve stress, provide physical assistance, and meet any special needs.

- Feelings of guilt are normal and common among caregivers. You have a hard and demanding job. When you feel guilty, ask yourself if doing more is really necessary or possible. Accept your limits.

- If things become overwhelming, consider talking to a counselor. A counselor can provide individual or family counseling about how to adjust to the changes Parkinson's is making in your life. (📖 See *Resources for APDA's, Caring for the Caregiver: Body, Mind, and Spirit.*)

> **Tip**
>
> Allow yourself to find the humor in caregiving and maintain regular contact with friends who are upbeat. Laugh heartily. Many people are not comfortable joking in front of someone who is ill. But providing a humorous setting may allow the person in your care to "forget" about their condition—if only for a short time.

> **NOTE**
>
> The person with PD is grieving over losses caused by PD and may be angry. Rude or offensive behavior should not be allowed. Bring these behaviors to the attention of the doctor to find out if they are medication symptoms.

Long-Distance Caregiving

Often the children of the PD person do not live in the same town or even country as the person with Parkinson disease. They will have to play a caring role from a distance that is meaningful and realistic. Long-distance caring is more likely to occur during the early stages of PD when the person is less likely to be physically dependent on others. During this time, care will consist mainly of understanding and emotional support. For the person at a distance, consider the following ideas:

- An important part of long-distance caring is to remain in regular touch. If possible, set a special day and time to call.

- Send a surprise care package regularly or at least a card.

- Financial help may be of great assistance. Ask clearly if you can help out with money.

- Learn about the medications being taken and encourage the family to tell the doctor of changes and problems.

- During a visit, ask to go with the PD patient to a doctor's appointment. Mention the things you may have noticed about symptoms, especially wearing-off.

- Ask about the health of the primary caregiver. Encourage the caregiver to take care of his or her own health.

- Invite the PD patient to visit you in order to give the primary caregiver a break.

- Offer to pay for respite care.

Consider developing a plan in advance. List necessary tasks, share responsibilities, and consider the possibilities. For example:

- Who is going to provide the majority of care?

- How can living arrangements be changed in order to help the person with PD stay in his or her home?

- If outside resources are needed, does the person with PD have the financial means to pay for them?

Create a notebook that includes useful information such as the doctor's name, address, and phone number, the person's medication, legal documents, health insurance policies and a list of contact persons in case of an emergency. Make sure that several people know where this information is kept.

Try and keep in touch with people are who are in regular contact with the person with Parkinson disease, for example, neighbors and friends. Ask them to stop by weekly to make sure that everything is ok. It may be harder to see changes in the pattern of a person with Parkinson disease if you do not see them on a regular basis.

Knowing When to Seek Help

If you have been a caregiver for an extended period and have great difficulty coping, by all means seek professional counseling.

You need professional help with the burden when you:

- are using more alcohol than usual in order to relax
- are using too many prescription drugs
- have physical symptoms such as skin rashes, back-aches, or a lingering cold or flu
- are unable to focus or concentrate
- feel lethargic
- feel keyed up and on edge
- feel constant sadness
- feel intense fear and anxiety
- feel worthless and guilty
- are depressed for two weeks or more
- are having thoughts of suicide
- have been or are thinking about becoming physically violent toward the person you are caring for.

At times like these, it may be necessary to think about using paid or voluntary help for a short time until you have worked through these difficulties.

When Hostility Builds to the Breaking Point

You can control your emotions by releasing anger and frustration in a safe way.

- Take a walk to cool down.
- Write your thoughts in a journal.
- Go to a private corner and unleash your anger on a big pillow.

Where to Find Professional Help or Support-Group Counseling

- the community pages of the phone directory
- the local county medical society, which can provide a list of counselors, psychologists, and psychiatrists
- community health clinics
- clergy or rabbi or other religious leader
- Area Agency on Aging
- online caregiver chat rooms
- United Way's "First Call for Help"
- a hospital's social service department
- a newspaper's calendar of support group meetings
- parish nurses

Ask for a counselor familiar with the needs of caregivers.

Letting Friends Help

If your friends want to know how they can help ease your burden, tell them to

- telephone and be a good listener as you may voice strong feelings
- offer words of appreciation for your efforts
- share a meal
- help you find useful information about community resources

Checklist **Dealing with Physical and Emotional Burdens**

✓ Do not allow the person in your care to take unfair advantage of you by being overly demanding.

✓ Live one day at a time.

✓ List priorities, decide what to leave undone, and think of ways to make the work easier.

✓ When doing a long, boring care task, use the time to relax or listen to music.

✓ Find time for regular exercise to increase your energy (even if you only stretch in place).

✓ Focus on getting relaxing sleep rather than more sleep.

✓ Set aside time for prayer or reflection.

✓ Practice deep breathing and learn to meditate to empty your mind of all troubles.

✓ Allow your self-esteem to rise because you have discovered hidden skills and talents.

✓ Realize your own limitations and accept them.

✓ Make sure your goals are realistic—you may be unable to do everything you could do before.

✓ Keep your eating habits balanced—do not fall into a toast-and-tea habit.

✓ *Take time for yourself.*

✓ *Treat yourself to a massage.*

✓ *Keep up with outside friends and activities.*

✓ *Spread the word that you would welcome some help, and allow friends to help with respite care.*

✓ *Delegate (assign) jobs to others. Keep a list of tasks you need to have done and assign specific ones when people offer to help.*

✓ *Share your concerns with a friend.*

✓ *Join a support group, or start one (to share ideas and resources).*

✓ *Use respite care when needed.*

✓ *Express yourself openly and honestly with people you feel should be doing more to help.*

✓ *When you visit your own doctor, be sure to explain your caregiving responsibilities, not just your symptoms.*

✓ *Allow yourself to feel your emotions without guilt. They are natural and very human.*

✓ *Unload your anger and frustration by writing it down.*

✓ *Allow yourself to cry and sob.*

✓ *Know that you are providing a very important service to the person in your care.*

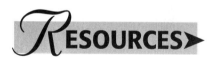

- show genuine interest

- stop by or send cards, letters, pictures, or humorous newspaper clippings

- share the workload

- help hire a relief caregiver

Remind you of saying, "Grant me the serenity to accept the things I cannot change, the courage to change the things I can, and the wisdom to know the difference."

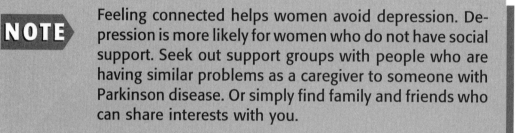

NOTE Feeling connected helps women avoid depression. Depression is more likely for women who do not have social support. Seek out support groups with people who are having similar problems as a caregiver to someone with Parkinson disease. Or simply find family and friends who can share interests with you.

$\mathcal{R}$ESOURCES➤

For more information on the material presented in this chapter, and free brochures on all topics related to Parkinson disease, contact:

American Parkinson Disease Association (APDA)
(800) 223-2732
www.apdaparkinson.org

European Parkinson's Disease Association (EPDA)
www.epda.eu.com

National Parkinson Foundation (NPF)
(800) 327-4545
www.parkinson.org

CAPS (Children of Aging Parents)
1609 Woodbourne Road, Suite 302A
Levittown, PA 19057-1511
(800) 227-7294
www.caps4caregivers.org
A nonprofit organization of caregiver support with groups, resources, and information.

Caregiver.com
www.caregiver.com
Maintains one of the most visited caregiver sites on the Internet, publishes Today's Caregiver Magazine. *Provides links to many resources such as government and non-profit agencies.*

Caregiver Survival Resources
www.caregiver911.com
A comprehensive list linking caregiving information and services for general issues and specific chronic illnesses.

Caring for the Caregiver: Body, Mind, and Spirit (APDA Educational Supplement No. 4). Available from the American Parkinson Disease Association.
(800) 223-2732

Center for Family Caregivers/Tad Publishing Co.
www.caregiving.com or www.familycaregivers.org
Develops and distributes educational materials on caregiving, including an electronic newsletter. Caregiving informational kits are $5 each; please specify new, seasoned, or transitioning caregiver when requesting a kit.

Eldercare Locator
(800) 677-1116
www.eldercare.gov
Finds adult protective services in your area for someone experiencing domestic violence. Locates other local resources providing services to elderly persons.

The Fine Art of "Re-Creation and Socialization" with Parkinson's Disease is available by calling the American Parkinson Disease Association.
(800) 223-2732
www.apdaparkinson.org
E-mail: info@apdaparkinson.org

Lotsa Helping Hands
www.lotsahelpinghands.com
Provides a free-of-charge Web service that allows family, friends, neighbors, and colleagues—the community circle—to assist more easily with daily meals, rides, shopping, and errands that may become a burden during times of medical crisis.

National Alliance for Caregivers
4720 Montgomery Lane, 5th Floor
Bethesda, MD 20184
www.caregiving.org
The Alliance is a non-profit coalition of national organizations focusing on issues of family caregiving.

National Family Caregivers Association
10400 Connecticut Avenue, Suite 500
Kensington, MD. 20895-2504
(800) 896-3650; (301) 942-6430; Fax: (301) 942-2302
www.nfcacares.org
E-mail: info@nfcacares.org
Publishes a member newsletter at no charge for family caregivers. Dues are $40 for professionals, $60 for nonprofits, and $100 for for-profit organizations.

Today's Caregiver Magazine
6365 Tuft Street, Suite 3003
Hollywood, FL 33024
(800) 829-2734
www.caregiver.com/magazine
Bimonthly magazine dedicated to caregivers.

Well Spouse Association
63 West Main Street, Suite H
Freehold, NJ 07728
(800) 838-0879
www.wellspouse.org
info@wellspouse.org
Publishes Mainstay, a bimonthly newsletter, and provides networking local support groups.

Check with your local church or health facility to see if they sponsor **"Share the Care"** teams.

Publications

Always on Call: When Illness Turns Families Into Caregivers by Carol Levine (ed.). 2000, United Hospital Fund.

Care for the Family Caregiver: A Place to Start, a report prepared by HIP Health Plan of new York and National Alliance for Caregiving. Available at www.caregiving.org

A Caregiver's Survival Guide: How to Stay Healthy When Your Loved One Is Sick by Kay Marshall Strom. 2000, Intervarsity Press.

Caring for Yourself While Caring for Others: A Caregiver's Survival and Renewal Guide by Lawrence Brammer and Marian Bingea. 1999, Vantage Press.

Caring for Yourself While Caring for Your Aging Parents: How to Help, How to Survive by Claire Berman. 1996, Henry Holt & Co.

The Complete Eldercare Planner by Joy Loverde. 2000, Three Rivers Press.

The Emotional Survival Guide for Caregivers by Barry J. Jacobs, PhD. 2006, The Guilford Press.

The Fearless Caregiver: How to Get the Best of Care for Your Loved One and Still Have a Life of Your Own by Gary Barg. 2001, Capital Books.

Helping Yourself Help Others: A Book for Caregivers by Rosalynn Carter, with Susan Golant. 1995, Random House/Time Books.

Love, Honor, and Value: A Family Caregiver Speaks Out About the Choices and Challenges of Caregiving by Susan Geffen Mintz. 2002, Capital Books.

Mainstay: For the Well Spouse of the Chronically Ill by Maggie Strong. 1997, Bradford Books.

Positive Caregiver Attitudes by James Sherman, PhD. 1996, Pathway Books.

Taking Care of Aging Family Members by Wendy Lustbader. 1994, Free Press.

Taking Time for Me: How Caregivers Can Effectively Deal with Stress by Katharine Karr.

Online Publications

Care Directions—The Internet's Complete Guide to Care and the Rights of the Elderly in the UK
www.caredirections.co.uk

Caregiver Survival Resources
www.caregiver911.com

The Caregivers Handbook
www.acsu.buffalo.edu/~drstall/hndbk0.html

The One-Stop Shop for All You Need to Know about Dysphagia and Swallowing Difficulties
www.dysphagianonline.com

Parkinson's Disease: Caring and Coping
www.parkinson.org/care4.htm

The Parkinson Patient at Home
www.cnsonline.org/www/archive/parkins/park-02.html

If you don't have home access to the Internet, ask your local library to help you locate any Web site.

Activities of Daily Living

*I*n this chapter you will learn how and when to provide physical assistance to the person in your care. As PD progresses and symptoms get worse, someone who used to be able to perform activities of daily living such as dressing, grooming, eating and toileting may now need assistance. Your daily activities may need to change.

As your everyday tasks change, you may need to cut back or cut out some activities such as housekeeping and caring for other family members. Caregivers may think they know what the person with PD needs or wants, but it is always better to ask. (📖 *See Resources* for APDA's, Helping Your Partner: What Not to Do!)

Personal Hygiene

As a caregiver, some of your time each day will be spent helping the person in your care with personal hygiene. This includes bathing, shampooing, oral or mouth care, shaving, and foot care.

Tip | **SKIN CARE**
It is easier to prevent chapping than to heal chapped skin, so apply lotion often.

NOTE ▷ Always start washing at the cleanest area and work toward the dirtiest area.

Tip Give a back rub with good-quality lotion to improve circulation. Avoid lanolin, which can dry the skin.

Tip Trim the toenails if they are long. If toenails are too thick, some podiatrists will make house calls for nail trims only. Medicare covers the cost in some states.

NOTE A build-up of earwax may make it hard for the person to hear. Have the ears checked and cleaned by a nurse or doctor twice a year. If the doctor approves, apply a little lotion to the outside of the ears to prevent drying and itching.

The Basin Bath

If the person in your care can be in a chair or wheelchair, you can give a sponge bath at the sink.

1. Make sure the room is warm.

2. Gather supplies—disposable gloves, mild soap, washcloth, washbasin, lotion, comb, electric razor, shampoo—and clean clothes.

3. Use good body mechanics (position)—keep your feet apart, stand firmly, bend your knees, and keep your back in a neutral position.

4. Offer the urinal.

5. Wash the face first.

6. Wash the rest of the upper body.

7. If the person can stand, wash the genitals. If the person is too weak to stand, wash the lower part of the body in the bed.

> **NOTE** Bathing three times a week is advised by dermatologists. Daily bathing is hard on older skin.

The Tub Bath

If the person in your care has good mobility and is strong enough to get in and out of the tub, he or she may enjoy a tub bath. Be sure there are grab bars, a bath bench, and a rubber mat so the person doesn't slide. (It may be easier to sit at bench level rather than at the bottom of the tub.) Use the following steps:

1. Make sure the room is warm.

2. Gather supplies—disposable gloves for the caregiver, mild soap, washcloth, lotion, comb, electric razor, shampoo—and clean clothes.

3. Check the water temperature before the person gets in.

4. Guide the person into the tub. Have the person use the grab bars. (Don't let the person grab you and pull you down.)

5. Help the person wash.

6. Empty the tub and then help the person get out.

7. Guide the person to use the grab bars while getting out. **OR**, have the person stand up and then sit on the bath bench. First swing one of the person's legs and then the other over the edge of the tub. Help the person stand.

8. Put a towel on a chair or the toilet lid and have the person sit there to dry off.

9. Apply lotion to any skin that appears dry.

10. Help the person dress.

Tip

BATHING IN THE TUB

If a bath bench is not used, many people feel more secure if they turn onto their side and then get on their knees before rising from the tub. This is a very helpful way to get out of the tub if the person is unsteady.

NOTE

Because tub baths can be difficult and risky for people with PD, showering is preferred. Using wash mitts (terry-cloth gloves) is better than holding a washcloth. A suction brush for grooming will reduce the chance of falls.

The Shower

Some people with PD (and older people) also have dementia (confusion). They can become frightened by the sound and feel of running water. It may be soothing to let the person smell the soap and feel the towel. Be sure the shower floor is not slippery. For safety's sake, be sure there are well-placed grab bars.

1. Make sure the room is warm.

2. Explain to the person what you are going to do.

3. Provide a shower stool in case the person needs to sit.

4. Gather supplies—mild soap, washcloth, washbasin, comb, electric razor, shampoo—and clean clothes.

5. To prevent burns, turn the cold water on first and then the hot. Test and adjust the water temperature before the person gets in. Use gentle water pressure.

6. First, spray and clean the less sensitive parts of the body such as the feet.

7. For safety, ask the person to hold the grab bar or sit on the shower stool.

8. Move the water hose around the person rather than asking the person to move.

9. Assist in washing as needed.

10. Guide the person out of the shower and wrap with a towel; then turn off the water.

11. Apply lotion to skin that appears dry.

12. If necessary, have the person sit on a stool or on the toilet lid.

13. Assist in drying and dressing.

For more tips on how to make showering easier, see *Resources for NPF's, Caring and Coping.*

> **NOTE** Remove from the bathing area any electrical equipment that could get wet.

Nail Care

When providing nail care, you can watch for signs of irritation or infection. This is especially important in a person with diabetes, where a small infection can turn into something more serious. Fingernails and toenails can thicken with age, which will make them more difficult to trim.

1. Assemble supplies—soap, basin with water, towel, nailbrush, scissors, nail clippers, file, and lotion.

2. Wash your hands.

3. Wash the hands of the person in your care with soap and water and soak the hands in a basin of warm water for 5 minutes.

4. Gently scrub the nails with the brush to remove trapped dirt.

5. Dry the nails and gently push back the cuticle (the skin around the nails) with the towel. Never cut the cuticle.

6. To prevent ingrown nails, cut fingernails and toenails straight across.

7. File gently to smooth the edges.

8. Gently massage the person's hands and feet with lotion.

NOTE If other members of the household are using the same equipment, clean the nail clippers with alcohol.

Shampooing the Hair

People with PD and older people may have difficulty shampooing their own hair in the shower. Keeping the hair and scalp clean improves blood flow to the scalp and keeps the hair healthy. Shampooing can be done anytime the person is not overly tired. The most convenient time may be right before a bath. Use a system that is easiest for you and the person in your care.

NOTE Hair must be rinsed thoroughly to avoid certain scalp conditions that are common in people with PD (dandruff, or seborrheic dermatitis). You may wish to use a shampoo that contains a mild coal tar or salicylic acid, like Neutrogena® or Ionil®.

Tip SHAMPOOING
To make washing easy, dilute the shampoo in a bottle before pouring it on the hair.

Wet Shampoo

1. Assemble supplies—latex gloves, comb and brush, shampoo/conditioner, several pitchers of warm water, large basin, washcloth, towels.

2. Have the person sit on a chair or commode.

3. Drape a large towel over the person's shoulders.

4. Gently comb any knots out of the hair.

5. Protect the person's ears with cotton.

6. Ask the person to cover his or her eyes with a washcloth and to lean over the sink.

7. Moisten the hair with a wet washcloth or with water poured from a pitcher.

8. Massage a small amount of diluted shampoo into the hair.

9. Remove the shampoo with clean water or a washcloth until the rinse water or cloth runs clear.

10. Use a leave-in conditioner if desired.

11. Towel dry the hair.

12. Remove the cotton from the person's ears.

13. Comb the hair gently.

14. If desired, use a hair dryer on the cool setting to dry hair. Be very careful not to burn the scalp.

OR

1. Cut a round slit at the raised edge of a heavy rubber dish-draining mat so that the end can tuck under

the person's neck and the water can drain down into the sink.

2. Seat the person at the kitchen sink with his or her back to the mat.

3. Place a towel on the person's shoulders. Place the rubber dish-draining mat with the round cut against the neck and the smooth edge draining into the sink (beauty salon style).

4. Follow the method for shampooing as above, using the sink hose or a pitcher to wash and rinse the hair.

Dry Shampoo

1. Assemble supplies—latex gloves for the caregiver, comb and brush, waterless shampoo, and towels.

2. Lather the head until all foam disappears.

3. Towel the hair dry and gently comb it.

 You can buy waterless shampoo from the pharmacy or at a medical supply company.

Wet Shampoo in Bed

1. Assemble supplies—latex gloves, comb and brush, shampoo/ conditioner, several pitchers of warm water, a large basin, plastic sheet, washcloth, towels, and hair dryer.

2. If possible, raise the bed.

3. Help the person lie flat.

4. Protect the bedding with plastic under the head and shoulders.

5. Roll the edges of the plastic inward so the water will run down into a basin placed on a chair next to the head of the bed.

6. Drape a towel over the person's shoulders.

7. Protect the person's ears with cotton.

8. Cover the person's eyes with a washcloth.

9. Moisten the hair with a wet washcloth.

10. Massage a small amount of diluted shampoo into the hair.

11. Remove the shampoo with a wet washcloth until the rinse water or water from the cloth runs clear.

12. Use a leave-in conditioner if desired.

13. Towel dry the hair.

14. Remove the cotton from the person's ears.

15. Comb the hair gently.

16. Use a hair dryer on the cool setting to dry hair. Be very careful not to burn the scalp.

EASIER SHAMPOOING
An enema bag attached to an IV pole provides an easy hose for shampooing.

Shaving

Some people prefer a wet shave with a safety razor. However, it may be safer for a person with PD to use an electric razor. (Growing a beard is one way to avoid this problem!)

Shaving can be done by the person in your care, or you can shave his whiskers with a safety razor or an electric razor. If he wears dentures, make sure they are in his mouth.

1. Assemble supplies—disposable gloves, safety razor, shaving cream, washcloth, towel, lotion.

2. Wash your hands.

3. Adjust the light so that you can clearly see his face but it is not shining in his eyes.

4. Spread a towel under his chin.

5. Soften the beard by wetting the face with a warm, damp washcloth.

6. Apply shaving cream to his face, carefully avoiding the eyes.

7. Hold the skin tight with one hand and shave in the direction the hair grows, using short firm strokes.

8. Be careful of sensitive areas.

9. Rinse the skin with a wet washcloth.

10. Pat his face dry with the towel.

11. Apply lotion if the skin appears dry.

NOTE Never use an electric razor if the person is receiving oxygen.

Oral Care

Oral care includes cleansing the mouth and gums and the teeth or dentures. Medications can cause dry mouth and less saliva. This may make the person with PD more at risk for tooth decay and for gum and bone disease. Prevention requires frequent brushing and flossing. Use an electric toothbrush if possible. There are floss holders available in drug stores that make it easier to floss. If the person with PD has dry mouth or gets sores from dentures, ask the pharmacist for saliva substitutes to use as an oral rinse.

Daily dental hygiene is important but can cause anxiety in some people. Always be patient and tell the person what you are about to do. (The person who refuses to brush can swish and spit out a fluoride mouthwash rinse.)

1. Gather supplies—disposable gloves, a soft toothbrush, toothpaste, baking soda, warm water in a glass, dental floss, and a bowl.

2. Bring the person to an upright position.

3. If possible, allow the person to clean his or her own teeth. This should be done twice daily and after meals.

4. Be sure the person can spit out water before allowing a sip. Use a water glass for rinsing.

5. If necessary, ask the person to open his or her mouth. Gently brush the front and back teeth up and down.

6. Rinse well by having the person sip water and spit into a bowl.

Denture Cleaning

1. Remove the dentures from the mouth.

2. Run them under water and soak them in cleaner in a denture cup.

3. Rinse the person's mouth with water or mouthwash.

4. Stimulate the gums with a very soft toothbrush.

5. Return the dentures to the person's mouth.

NOTE Even a person with dentures should regularly visit the dentist to check the soft tissues of the mouth.

Foot Care

For the comfort and good health of the person in your care:

• Provide properly fitting low-heeled shoes with Velcro® or elastic closures and nonslip soles. Avoid shoes with heavy soles, running shoes with rubber tips over the toes, and shoes with thick cushioning, which can make an older person fall.

- Provide cotton socks rather than acrylic.
- Trim the person's nails only after a bath when they have softened.
- Use a disposable sponge-tipped toothbrush to clean or dry between the toes.
- Check feet daily for bumps, cuts, and red spots.

Call the doctor or other health care provider if a sore develops on the foot. A person with diabetes must have special foot care to prevent infections. Infections may result in the amputation of a foot.

Common Leg and Foot Problems and Solutions

Problem	Solution
Foot strain	Visit a podiatrist.
Calluses	Rub emollient lotion or cream on the area; do not cut hard skin.
Cramps	Relieve by movement and massage.
Hammer toes and bunions	Wedge a pad between the big toe and the second toe to straighten them; cut holes in the shoe to relieve rubbing.
Leg ulcers (openings in the skin)	Follow the doctor's instructions. Exercise to keep the foot and ankle mobile.
Swollen legs or ankles	Follow the doctor's instructions for treatment of the underlying cause. In some forms of PD, swollen ankles are present and misinterpreted as signs of congestive heart failure.
Varicose veins	Elevate the legs twice a day for 30 minutes. Before lowering the legs, apply an elastic bandage or stocking.

> **NOTE** Foot pain can cause a person to lean back on his or her heels and increase the chance of a fall, so keep toenails trimmed and feet healthy.

Dressing

Dressing will take longer than usual because of declining motor skills and loss of strength. Pain and stiffness in the limbs can make it more difficult to put on or take off clothing, especially underwear, socks, and pants. DO NOT RUSH the person while dressing. Allow the person to do as much alone as he or she can, using special aids. (📖 See *Equipment and Supplies,* p. 92.)

Dressing Someone with PD

- Always allow plenty of time to dress so that you do not feel rushed. You may find it easier to do things like buttons while sitting in a chair with arm rests.

- Choose clothes that can be slipped on easily, such as simple dresses, jumpers, or pants with elastic waists, and shoes with Velcro. Dressing a person with disabilities can be made easier by setting up a routine. Before you begin, lay the clothes out in the order they will be put on.

- Dress the person while he or she is sitting.

- Use adaptive equipment (dressing aids) like a button-hook and shoehorn. (📖 See *Equipment and Supplies*, p. 93.)

- Avoid clothes with busy patterns. They may make it more difficult for the person to find buttons and zippers.

- Use loose clothes that are easy to put on and have elastic waistbands, Velcro® fasteners, and front openings.

- Use bras with front closures.

- Half-ankle socks are easier to pull on.

- For a person who cannot get out of bed, use a gown with a back closure (for ease of opening when using a bedpan or urinal).

NOTE For a bedridden person, be sure to smooth out all wrinkles in the clothes and bedding. This will help prevent pressure sores.

Sitting, Standing, Walking

- If sitting down or getting up is difficult for the person in your care, choose a high, straight-backed chair with arms. Avoid having deep, soft armchairs or settees.

- Have the person stand still for a few seconds after rising to regain balance.

- If the person becomes "frozen" in place, tell the person to rock gently from side to side or pretend he or she is stepping over an object on the floor.

- Physiotherapy (physical therapy) and other complementary therapies can provide exercises that will assist with balance and walking.

Bed Making

Making a bed with someone in it will be easier if you follow these steps:

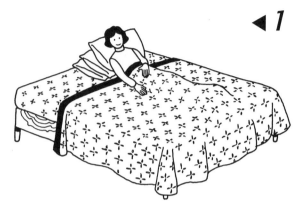

◀ **1**

- The bed has two parts—the side the person is lying on and the side you are making.

- If you have a hospital bed, raise the height of the bed.

- Lower the head and foot of the bed so that it is flat.

Draw sheet

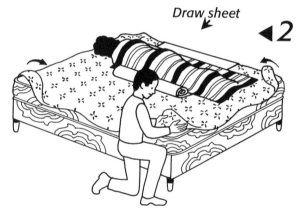

◀ **2**

- Loosen the sheets on all sides.

- Remove the blankets and pillow, leaving only the bottom and top sheets.

- Cover the person with a bath blanket (a flannel sheet or large towel) for modesty and warmth.

- Pull the top sheet out from under the bath blanket.

- Raise the bed rail on the side across from you (the opposite side) so the person cannot fall out of bed. If you don't have a hospital bed, be sure the bed is pushed against the wall.

- Roll the person over to the opposite side of the bed.

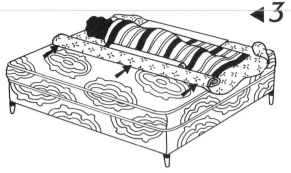

◄ **3**
- Roll all the old bottom sheeting toward the person.

Clean sheet

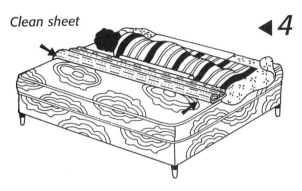

◄ **4**
- Fold the clean sheet, along with other mattress covers, lengthwise.
- Place it on the bed with the middle fold running along the center of the mattress right beside the person's body.

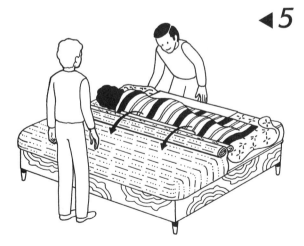

◄ **5**
- Unfold the clean sheet and bring enough of it toward you to cover half of the bed.
- Gently lift the mattress and tuck the sheet in.
- Tuck the free edge of the draw sheet under the mattress on your side of the bed.
- Ask the person to roll over the linens in the middle of bed to the clean side.

OR

- Bend as close to the person's body as possible. Place your hand and arm under the person's shoulders and move the person and the bath blanket over the linens in the center of the bed.

- If it is a hospital bed, raise the bed rail on your side and lock it into place.

- Go to the other side and remove all soiled linen. Tuck in all the linen and pull tight on the sheets to remove all wrinkles so they don't rub and irritate the person's skin.

- Change the pillowcase.

- Spread the top sheet over the person and bath blanket.

- Ask the person to hold the sheet while you pull the bath blanket away.

- Tuck the sheet under the mattress at the foot of the bed.

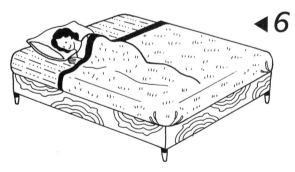

◀ 6
- Spread a blanket over the top. (The blanket should be up far enough to cover the person's shoulders.)

- Fold the sheet down over the blanket.

- Adjust the person in bed so she is comfortable.

Toileting

Always wear latex gloves when helping with toileting. This prevents the spread of disease. Wash your hands before and after providing care.

Toileting in Bed

When a person is mobile, toileting in bed should not be encouraged.

Toileting in Bed for a Female or for Bowel Movements

1 • Warm the bedpan with warm water. Empty the water into the toilet.

• Powder the bedpan with talcum powder to keep the skin from sticking to it.

• Place a tissue or water in the pan to make cleaning easier. Or use a light spray of vegetable oil in the bedpan, which will make it easier to empty the contents.

• Raise the person's gown.

◄*2* • Ask the person to raise her hips.

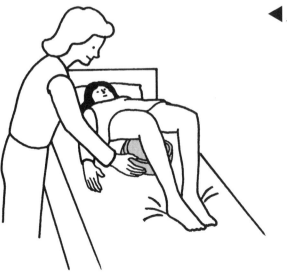

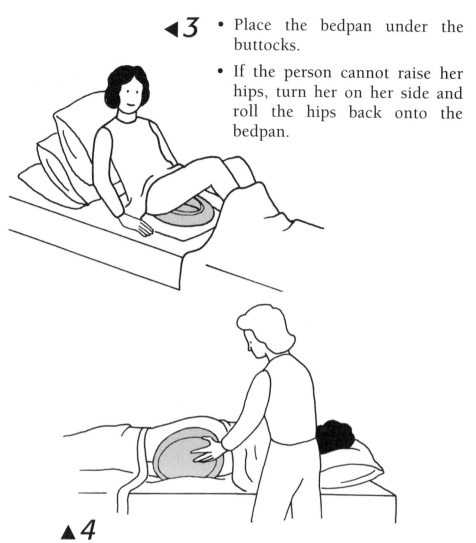

◀ **3**
- Place the bedpan under the buttocks.

- If the person cannot raise her hips, turn her on her side and roll the hips back onto the bedpan.

▲ **4**

- If the person cannot do so, clean the anal area with bathroom tissue. Then use a wet tissue to clean the area.

- After the woman has urinated, pour a cup of warm water over her genitals and pat the area dry with a towel.

- Wash the person's hands.

- Remove and empty the bedpan.

- Be sure to wash your hands.

Using a Urinal

1. If the person can't do so himself, place the penis into the urinal as far as possible and hold it in.

2. When the person signals he is finished, remove and empty the urinal.

3. Wash his hands.

4. Wash your own hands.

Using a Commode

A portable commode is helpful for a person with limited mobility. The portable commode (with the pail removed) can be used over the toilet seat and as a shower seat.

Using a Portable Commode

1. Gather the portable commode, toilet tissue, a basin, a cup of water, a washcloth or paper towel, soap, and a towel.

2. Wash your hands.

3. Help the person onto the commode.

4. Offer toilet tissue.

5. Pour a cup of warm water on female genitalia.

6. Pat the area dry with a paper towel.

7. Offer a washcloth so the person can wash the hands.

8. Remove the pail from under the seat, empty it, rinse it with clear water, and empty the water into the toilet.

9. Wash your hands.

Tip

TOILET SAFETY
Use Velcro® with tape on the back. Attach it to the back of the toilet or commode seat to keep the lid from falling.

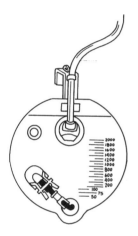

Using the Bathroom Toilet

If the mobile person is missing the toilet, get a toilet seat in a color that is different from the color of the floor. This may help him see the toilet better. If he is failing to cleanse the anal area, or failing to wash his hands, use tact to encourage him to do so. This will help prevent the spread of infections.

Catheters

A urinary catheter is a device made from rubber or plastic that drains urine from the body. It is inserted by a nurse through the urethra (a tube that connects the bladder to the outside of the body) into the bladder (an organ that collects urine).

A Foley catheter stays in the bladder and drains into a bag attached to a person's leg, the bed, or a chair. When caring for someone with this kind of catheter (called an indwelling catheter), watch for these things:

1. Be sure the tube stays straight and drains properly. Check for kinks in the tubing.

2. Be sure the level of urine in the bag increases.

3. Be sure the drainage bag is always lower than the bladder.

4. Use tape or straps when securing a catheter to someone's inner thigh.

5. In males, an erection is a common reaction to the catheter.

6. Tell the doctor if blood or sediment (matter that settles to the bottom) appears in the tubing or bag.

NOTE A Foley catheter greatly increases the risk of infection. It is chosen as a last resort to manage incontinence.

Care of the Person Who Has a Catheter

1. Wash your hands.

2. Put on gloves.

3. Position the person on his or her back.

4. Take care not to pull on the catheter.

5. While holding the catheter, wash the area around it with a washcloth.

6. To avoid infection, wipe toward the anus, not back and forth.

NOTE To prevent foul odors due to the growth of bacteria in the urine drainage bag, put a few drops of hydrogen peroxide in the bag when it is emptied.

Changing a Catheter from Straight Drainage to Leg Bag

1. Gather supplies—disposable gloves, a bed protector, alcohol wipes, and a leg bag with straps.

2. Uncover the end of the catheter and draining tubing; put a towel or other bed protector under this area.

3. Disconnect the drainage tubing from the catheter.

4. Wipe the attachment tube of the leg bag with an alcohol swab and insert it into the catheter.

5. Place the cap attached to the urinary drainage bag over the end of the tubing to keep it clean and prevent urine from leaking out.

6. Secure the tubing to the person's leg.

Condom Catheter

The doctor may prescribe a condom catheter for a male if infections from an indwelling catheter become a chronic problem. The catheter fits over the penis like a condom. Leakage is often a problem with this type of aid. **It is extremely important that a condom catheter not be secured too tightly, which can result in serious injury.**

Incontinence

Incontinence is the involuntary leakage of urine or a bowel movement over which the person has no control. It is a symptom, not a disease, and should never be considered as a normal part of aging or illness. It can be caused by stroke, multiple sclerosis, infection, vaginitis, injury to the pelvic region, diseases involving brain cells or nerves to the bladder, or willful incontinence due to laziness and confusion. Treatments include bladder training, exercises to strengthen the pelvic floor (Kegel exercises), biofeedback, surgery, electrical muscle conditioner, urinary catheter, prosthetic devices, or external collection devices. Talk to the doctor about the options or treatments for the person in your care.

To Manage Incontinence:

- Avoid alcohol, coffee, spicy foods, and citrus foods. This can irritate the bladder and can cause sudden urination.

- Give fluids at regularly spaced times to dilute the urine. This decreases the irritation of the bladder.

- Be sure the person in your care voids (goes to the bathroom) regularly (ideally every 2 hours). Use an alarm clock to keep track of the time.

- Provide clothing that can be easily removed.

- Keep a bedpan or a portable commode in or near the bed.

- Provide absorbent products (adult diapers) to be worn under clothes.
- Stroke or tap the lower abdomen to cause voiding.
- Keep the skin dry and clean. Urine on the skin can cause pressure sores and infection.
- Your patience and understanding will help the person have confidence and self-respect.

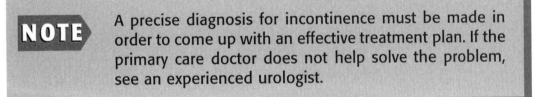

NOTE A precise diagnosis for incontinence must be made in order to come up with an effective treatment plan. If the primary care doctor does not help solve the problem, see an experienced urologist.

Urinary Tract Infection

Urinary tract infection may be present if the person has

- blood in the urine
- a burning feeling when voiding
- cloudy urine with sediment (matter that settles to the bottom)
- cramping in the lower abdomen or side
- fever and chills
- foul-smelling urine
- a frequent, strong urge to void or frequent voiding
- pain in the lower back

Call the doctor if there are any signs of a urinary tract infection.

Bowel Hygiene: Optimal Bowel Function

The bowel becomes sluggish as we grow older; plus chronic neurological disorders such as Parkinson disease can further aggravate "gut" problems. Restoring optimal bowel function may require many weeks of establishing new habits, but is certainly worth the effort. Treatment goals include:

- weaning away from regular use of stimulant laxatives
- achieving spontaneous, soft stools 5–8 × per week
- avoiding hemorrhoids caused by straining-at-stool

Interventions

- Increase water consumption to 6–8 cups per day. Seltzer water adds air as well as moisture to the bowel, which can increase intestinal motility (stomach emptying).

- Reduce red meat and milk/dairy products in the diet. Increase fruits and vegetables.

- Increase weight-bearing exercise; try crawling or water exercises if poor balance prevents walking as exercise.

- Practice regular belly massage from the rib cage to the pubic bone.

- 6 oz. (3/4 cup) of hot tea or hot water with lemon juice on arising each morning can act as a bowel stimulant. Or try prune juice with pulp (*Sunsweet*).

- Stool softeners (*not* in combination with laxatives) such as *Colace, Equalactin,* or an Ayurvedic combination called *Triphala,* can be used regularly. Bulk/fiber additives (*Metamucil, Citrucel,* etc.) should *not* be used unless a minimum of 48 oz of water is consumed throughout the day.

- Infant-sized glycerin suppositories can aid in softening hard, dry stool in the lower colon. An occasional Fleet enema is OK if no stool is passed for 4–5 days or constipation is causing abdominal cramping.

NOTE Never sit on the toilet for longer than 5 minutes or strain to pass hard stool. Learn to honor your body's natural urges vs. attempting to produce a bowel movement "on schedule."

Tip Kathrynne Holden, RD, and author of *Eat Well, Stay Well with Parkinson Disease*, recommends the following recipe to manage constipation: Mix 1/2 cup applesauce, 2–4 tablespoons miller's bran, and 4–6 oz. prune juice (with or without pulp). Store in the refrigerator. Take a tablespoonful a day at first, gradually adding more if needed until you find the amount that works well for your person with PD. Prune juice is a natural laxative and softens the bran, and the applesauce sweetens the taste.

Diarrhea

Diarrhea (loose, watery stools) occurs when the intestines push stool along before the water in them can be reabsorbed (taken up) by the body. This condition can be caused by viral stomach flu, antibiotics, or stress anxiety.

To counteract diarrhea, consider two types of anti-diarrheals: those that thicken the stool, and those that slow intestinal spasms. Ask the pharmacist for advice.

Precautions:

- Do not use these treatments during the first 6 hours after diarrhea begins.

- Do not use if a fever is present.

- Stop giving the medications as soon as the stool thickens.

- Give plenty of fluids to prevent dehydration.

Diarrhea in people who are immobile is often caused by impaction. This is a blockage formed by hardened stool, with liquid stool passing around it. This must always be taken into consideration, because the usual treatments for diarrhea would be extremely dangerous if the diarrhea is being caused by impaction.

Hemorrhoids

Hemorrhoids are swollen, inflamed veins around the anus. They cause tenderness, pain, and bleeding. To treat hemorrhoids, you should do the following:

- Be sure to keep anal area clean with premoistened tissues.
- Apply zinc oxide or petroleum jelly to the area.
- Relieve itching by using cold compresses on the anus for 10 minutes several times a day.
- Ask the doctor about suppositories.

Call the Doctor:

- If blood from the hemorrhoids is dark red or brown and heavy
- If bleeding continues for more than one week
- If bleeding seems to occur for no reason

Control of Infection in the Home

Common health practices such as frequent hand-washing are necessary to avoid the risk of bacterial, viral, and fungal infections.

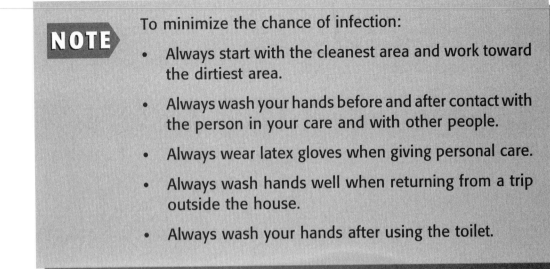

NOTE

To minimize the chance of infection:

- Always start with the cleanest area and work toward the dirtiest area.

- Always wash your hands before and after contact with the person in your care and with other people.

- Always wear latex gloves when giving personal care.

- Always wash hands well when returning from a trip outside the house.

- Always wash your hands after using the toilet.

Cleaning Techniques

The following techniques will help cut the chance of infection in the home.

Caregiver Hand-washing

- Hand-washing is the single most effective way to prevent the spread of infection or germs.

- Use antibacterial, bottle-dispensed soap.

- If the person in your care has an infection, use antimicrobial soap.

- Rub your hands for at least 30 seconds to produce lots of lather. Do this away from running water so that the lather is not washed away.

- Use a nailbrush on your nails; keep nails trimmed.

- Wash front and back of hands, between fingers, and at least 2 inches up your wrists.

- Repeat the process.

- Dry your hands on a clean towel or a paper towel.

Precautions for Anyone Who Pushes His or Her Own Wheelchair

- Wear leather gloves.

- Wash your hands frequently.

- For frequent in-between washings, use packaged cleansing towelettes.

Handling Soiled Laundry

- Do not carry soiled linen close to your body.

- *Never* shake dirty items or put soiled linens on the floor. They can contaminate (infect) the floor, and germs will be spread throughout the house on the soles of shoes.

- Store infected soiled linen in a leak-proof plastic bag and tie it closed.

- Bag soiled laundry in the same place where it is used.

- Wash soiled linen separately from other clothes.

- Fill the machine with hot water, add bleach (no more than 1/4 cup) and detergent. Rinse twice, and then dry.

- Clean the washer by running it through a cycle with 1 cup of bleach or other disinfectant to kill germs.

- Use rubber gloves when handling soiled laundry.

- Wash your hands.

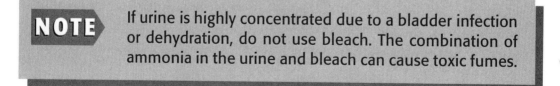

NOTE If urine is highly concentrated due to a bladder infection or dehydration, do not use bleach. The combination of ammonia in the urine and bleach can cause toxic fumes.

Disposal of Body Fluids

- Wear gloves (recommended for handling all body fluids).

- Flush liquid and solid waste down the toilet.
- Place used dressings and disposable (throwaway) pads in a sturdy plastic bag, tie securely, and place in a sealed container for collection.

Preventing Odors Caused by Bacteria

Bacteria need moisture, warm body temperature, oxygen, darkness, and nourishment to grow. Some strong odors may be eliminated by

- sprinkling baking soda on the wound dressing
- leaving an open can of finely ground coffee under the bed
- pouring a few drops of mouthwash in commodes and bedpans
- placing cotton balls soaked with mouthwash in the room
- spraying a fine mist of white distilled vinegar mixed with a few drops of eucalyptus or peppermint essential oil
- soaking cotton balls with vanilla extract and placing them in containers that retain strong odors
- using electrical and mechanical devices (such as fans, purifiers, and plug-in fresheners) to remove odor
- buying natural organic room sprays

Skin Care and Prevention of Pressure Sores

Pressure sores (also called decubiti or bedsores) are blisters or breaks in the skin. They are caused when the body's weight presses blood out of a certain area. The best treatment of pressure sores is prevention. How much time they take to heal depends on how advanced they are.

Facts

- The most common areas for sores are the bony areas—tailbone, hips, heels, and elbows.

- Sores can appear when the skin keeps rubbing on a sheet.

- The skin breakdown starts from the inside, works up to the surface, and can occur in just 15 minutes.

- Damage can range from a change in color in unbroken skin to deep wounds down to the muscle or bone.

- For people with light skin in the first stage of a bedsore, the skin color may change to a dark purple or red area that does not become pale under fingertip pressure. For people with dark skin, this area may become darker than normal.

- The affected area may feel warmer than the skin around it.

- Pressure sores that are not treated can lead to hospitalization and can require skin grafts.

Prevention

- Check the skin daily. (Bath time is the ideal time to do this.)

- Provide a well-balanced diet, with enough vitamin C, zinc, and protein.

- Keep the skin dry and clean. (Urine left on the skin can cause sores and infection.)

- Keep clothing loose.

- If splints or braces are used, make sure they are adjusted properly.

- Massage the body with light pressure, using equal parts surgical spirit and glycerin. (Ask a nurse or a pharmacist for advice.)

- If the person in your care sits in one chair for extended periods of time, put a gelfoam pad in the seat to reduce pressure on the tailbone.

- Turn a person who is unable to get out of bed at least every 2 hours. Change the person's positions. Smooth wrinkles out of sheets.

- Lightly tape foam to bony sections of the body using paper tape, which will not hurt the skin when peeled off.

- Use flannel or 100% cotton sheets to absorb moisture.

- Provide an egg-crate or sheepskin mattress pad for added comfort.

- Rent an electrically operated ripple bed. These beds have sections that can be inflated separately and at different times.

- Avoid using a plastic sheet or a Chux if they cause sweating.

- When the person is sitting, encourage changing the body position every 15 minutes.

- Use foam pads on chair seats to cushion the buttocks.

- Change the type of chair the person sits in; try using an open-back garden chair occasionally.

- Provide as much exercise as possible.

WOUND PREVENTION

If a person tends to scratch or pick at a spot, have the person wear cotton gloves. (Make sure the hands are clean and dry before putting the gloves on.)

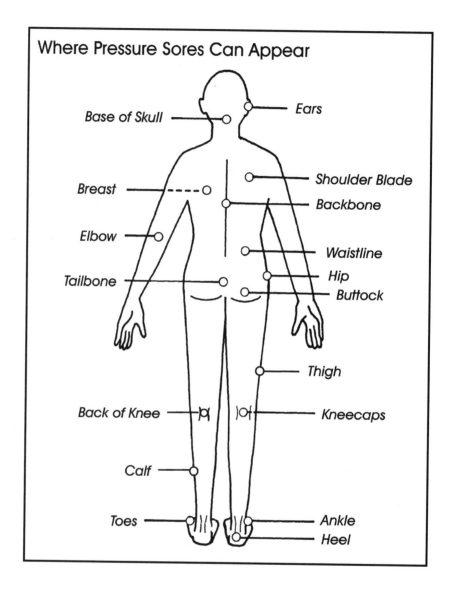

Where Pressure Sores Can Appear

Base of Skull

Ears

Breast

Shoulder Blade

Backbone

Elbow

Waistline

Tailbone

Hip

Buttock

Thigh

Back of Knee

Kneecaps

Calf

Toes

Ankle

Heel

Eating

The person with PD may take longer to eat. You may have to reheat food during the meal. Mealtimes are important times for people who are elderly or ill because they provide a welcome break in the day. If it is not too distracting for the person, include the family at mealtime. It is important that mealtimes are enjoyable so that eating is encouraged.

People who eat alone or who have disabilities may not be receiving proper nutrition. Look for these free or low-cost solutions:

Community meals—local meal programs at senior centers sponsored by the federal government and open to anyone over 59 and their spouses (call your local Area Agency on Aging or Department of Health and Human Resources)

Meals on Wheels—hot meals delivered to the home (call the Visiting Nurse Association)

Food stamps—provide help based on income that can stretch food dollars (call Department of Health and Human Resources or the Area Agency on Aging)

For best results at meal times:

- Allow 30 to 45 minutes for eating.
- Avoid fussy meal presentation.
- Make sure all items are ready to eat and within reach.
- Provide the same comfortable table and chair or other eating arrangement.
- Supply easy-to-hold eating utensils. To avoid cuts, throw out all chipped cups and plates.

- Reduce excess noise such as television and radio.
- If the person's vision is poor, place the same food on the same part of the plate every time.

Feeding Someone in Bed

NOTE Never offer food or drink to someone who is lying down.

1. Prop the head with pillows.
2. Provide an over-the-bed table.
3. Do not rush feeding, but maintain a steady pace.
4. Cut the food into bite-size portions, if necessary.
5. Explain what food is being served.
6. Fill cups only halfway.
7. Let the person hold the cup if he or she wants to. (A terry-cloth wristband slipped over the cup may make it easier to hold.)
8. Use available eating aids. (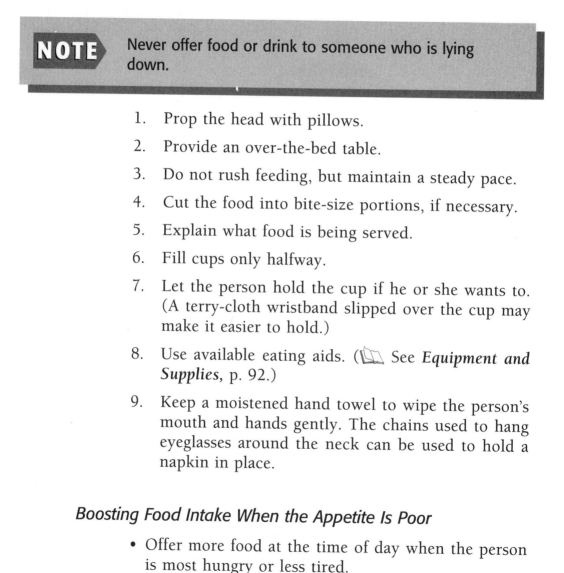 See *Equipment and Supplies,* p. 92.)
9. Keep a moistened hand towel to wipe the person's mouth and hands gently. The chains used to hang eyeglasses around the neck can be used to hold a napkin in place.

Boosting Food Intake When the Appetite Is Poor

- Offer more food at the time of day when the person is most hungry or less tired.
- Offer smaller, more frequent meals (see *Diet and Nutrition,* p. 199).

- Between meals, provide a nourishing snack, such as stewed fruit, tapioca pudding, or finger foods.

- To make food more appealing to those with decreased taste and smell, provide strong flavors.

- Add fat by using butter, margarine, or olive oil on foods.

- Add nonfat dry-milk powder to foods like yogurt, mashed potatoes, gravy, and sauces.

- Tell the person to eat with his or her fingers, if that is the only way to get the person to eat.

- Offer milk or fruit shakes.

- Pureed baby foods taste better in recent years and may be helpful.

(📖 See *Diet and Nutrition*, p. 201.)

NOTE ▷ If the person in your care needs to swallow three or four times with each bite of food; coughs before, during, or after swallowing; pockets food in the mouth; or senses something caught or sticking in the back of the throat, he or she may have a condition called dysphagia. Difficulty swallowing must be evaluated to determine if it is a symptom of a treatable condition and to help the caregiver learn proper feeding techniques.

Eating Problems and Solutions

Excessive repetition in swallowing/chewing—Coach the person to switch back and forth between hot and cold foods.

Difficulty chewing—Use denture adhesive and change the diet to soften foods.

Difficulty swallowing—Put foods through a blender or food mill; avoid thin liquids and instead serve thick liquids such as shakes or purees.

Poor scooping—Use bowls instead of plates or use swivel spoons.

Difficulty cutting food—Use a small pizza cutter or rolling knife.

Trouble moving food to the back of the mouth—Change the food's thickness and show the person how to direct the food to the center of the mouth.

Too dry or never dry mouth—This is often a side effect of antiparkinson medications.

Too easily distracted—Pull down the shades and remove the distractions.

Learn the Heimlich maneuver, which can help save the life of a choking person (☐ see *Emergencies,* p. 247).

> **NOTE** Difficulty swallowing can cause food or liquids to be taken into the lungs, which can lead to pneumonia. Reduce the chance of food entering the lungs by keeping the person upright for at least 20 minutes after a meal.

Speech and Swallowing

Many people with PD notice gradual changes in voice volume or the ability to speak clearly, which can be frustrating for both the person affected and the caregiver. The voice may become very soft or raspy, and consonants may sound slurred.

It helps to have the individual face the person he is talking to and make a deliberate attempt to speak louder.

This often sounds "fake" or too loud to the care receiver who is disbelieving of the quiet nature of his voice, but is just right for the listener struggling to understand.

A specialized speech therapy program called the *Lee Silverman Voice Treatment Method (LSVT)* has proven effective in treating speech problems common in Parkinson disease. Many speech–language pathologists (SLP) in the U.S. and some in other countries have taken the training to use the LSVT techniques.

LSVT focuses on one simple therapeutic target: increased vocal loudness. At the end of one month of treatment, which is often covered by Medicare and other insurers, patients are able to demonstrate dramatic improvement in functional communication skills. Quality of life can be considerably improved with this intensive but rather short-duration program. For more information or referral to an SLP trained in LSVT, go online to www.lsvt.org.

Singing is great exercise for the voice! Singing uses the same muscles that are used for speech. Encourage your person with PD to take a deep breath and join you in singing a favorite song. Encourage him to reach for the high and low notes and sing the lyrics with crisp, clear diction. This is not only a great breath-control exercise, but is a good emotional connection and just plain fun for both of you (see **Resources** *for NPF's, Speech and Swallowing*).

Swallowing Changes

People with PD may notice changes or difficulty with chewing, eating, or swallowing. These changes can happen at any time, but they tend to increase as PD progresses. Common changes include:

- Slowness in eating
- A sensation that food is caught in the throat
- Coughing or choking while eating or drinking

- Difficulty swallowing pills and drooling

- Drooling caused by a decrease in swallowing reflex.

Swallowing Evaluation

You can assess whether the person in your care has a swallowing problem by asking the following questions:

- Have you recently lost weight without trying?

- Do you avoid drinking liquids?

- Do you have the sensation that food is stuck in your throat?

- Do you drool at night? During the day?

- Does food collect around your gum line?

- Do you cough or choke before, during, or after eating or drinking?

- Do you often have heartburn or a sore throat?

- Do you have trouble moving food to the back of your mouth?

- Do you have trouble keeping food or liquid in your mouth?

- Does it take you a long time to eat a meal?

- Do you have trouble swallowing pills?

- Have your eating habits changed recently or have you had a loss of appetite?

- Do you sometimes have fever for no reasons?

- Do you notice changes in your voice after eating or drinking?

If the answer is "yes" to any of the questions, the person in your care may need to call a speech-language pathologist for a swallowing assessment. The physician or other health care provider can help you with a referral.

Swallowing Checklist

This form is to be completed by the caregiver about the person with PD. Think about each statement and check "yes" or "no" after each statement:

The person in my care:

❏ seems uninterested in food

❏ coughs or "strangles" during meals

❏ often coughs following a meal when we are doing other activities such as watching TV or reading

❏ takes longer to eat a meal than before

❏ sounds "wet" or "gurgly" when he or she speaks

❏ I have had to use the Heimlich maneuver on the person in my care.

Checked boxes are symptoms of chewing, swallowing, or eating difficulties. Seek referral for a swallowing evaluation by a qualified speech-language pathologist.

How to Improve Swallowing

The following tips and techniques can help the caregiver aid the person with PD to improve eating, chewing, and swallowing:

• Always have the person sit upright when eating, drinking, and taking pills.

• Give small amounts of food. Have the person chew well and swallow everything before giving more food.

• Have the person swallow twice after every bite.

• Put the fork down between bites to slow down the person's eating.

• Give small sips when providing a drink. Have the person take sips between each bite.

- Give only one sip at a time. Do not allow the person to gulp.

- Be careful when using straws. Straws are useful when someone has severe tremors or dyskinesias, but can put too much liquid too far back in the mouth too quickly.

- If using a straw, put it only in the front of the mouth.

- Keep the person's chin slightly down or at least parallel to the table. If the chin is raised, there is a risk of fluid getting into the lungs.

- Do not give a drink out of a can. Use a glass instead.

- Discourage the person in your care from talking with food in his or her mouth.

Certain types of foods can affect the chewing and swallowing of a person with PD. Raw vegetables, nuts, and peanut butter may be more difficult to chew or swallow. The best foods are moist, slippery, don't crumble or fall apart, and require less vigorous chewing. A speech-language pathologist or registered dietitian can suggest foods and drinks that are easiest to swallow. An occupational therapist can recommend various types of helpful tools that can make eating a more pleasant experience.

Drooling

Because of decreased frequency of swallowing, a person with PD may have more saliva pooled in the mouth than usual. Frequent sips of water or sucking on ice chips during the day can make the person swallow more often. Have the person keep the head up, chin parallel to the floor, and lips closed when not talking or eating. Sugar tends to make more saliva in the mouth, so reducing sugar intake can be helpful.

Many people with PD complain that they have a thick phlegm or mucus in the throat. Drinking more water will help thin the phlegm. Drinking carbonated beverages, such as soda, or tea with lemon may also help. Eating or drinking dairy products can make phlegm worse. (📖 See *Resources* for NPF's, *Speech & Swallowing* for more information.)

Cognitive Changes

Some people with Parkinson disease complain of slowness in thinking and difficulty finding the right words. When these cognitive (thinking) changes happen, the caregiver often will finish the person's sentences. Often, the person with PD will begin to avoid conversation. These mild changes are handled well by most people. Some patients actually report *improvements* in motivation and concentration when they take the dopaminergic medications used to treat Parkinson disease.

Dementia refers to cognitive changes that interfere with activities of daily living or affect the quality of life. A decrease in short-term memory plus at least one other area of cognitive dysfunction must exist before the medical term "dementia" is used. Of those people with PD who have dementia, it typically shows up long after the appearance of motor symptoms.

NOTE When dementia precedes motor symptoms or appears early on, it may signal a diagnosis other than PD.

Tip Fun for you and the person in your care—daily activities that involve movement to music (dancing, marching, singing, swaying).

Here are some ways to address cognitive changes:

- Try to preserve whatever skills the person has and help the person stay independent. Give no more assistance than is needed. Let the person help with whatever tasks he or she can still do.

- Break tasks down into small parts. For example, a meal is made up of sitting down at the table, picking up a fork, spearing the food, raising it to the mouth, etc.

- Set up a routine and stick to it.

- Avoid overstimulation. Pay attention to lighting, noise, and the number of people around.

- Provide visual cues. For instance, cabinet doors and drawers may be labeled with pictures and names of the contents.

- Improve the person's access to safe places and materials by using labels and pictures. Limit access to dangerous areas or materials by using latches or locks on doors, drawers, and cabinets.

- Don't assume that a behavior can't be changed. Always look for a treatable cause of the symptoms. Clues to watch for include pain, hunger, thirst, and medication side effects.

- If you can't figure out why a problem behavior continues, keep a log. Write down what happened before and after the behavior. This will help find links between cues, behavior, and rewards.

(📖 See **Resources** for NPF's, *Parkinson's Disease: Speaking Out*.)

Dealing with Memory Issues

Take care of the person's general health issues (high blood pressure, high cholesterol, diabetes), which can affect memory. Be on the lookout for urinary tract infections and lung infections. They can have a serious effect

on people with PD. Older peopl[...]
tory infections may not run a [...]

- When filling prescriptions, [...]

- Avoid falls and injuries, esp[...] and brain. Have the person u[...] walker, or wheelchair as ne[...]

- Sleep disorders are common [...] should avoid alcohol, tobacc[...] part of the day. (This does n[...] in the morning!) Reduce fluids in the later hours of the day. Be aware of medications wearing-off during sleep. Be careful about long-term use of sleep medications as they affect memory. Consider a sleep evaluation.

- Have the person's vision and hearing checked. A person with PD can't "remember" information if he or she hasn't heard it in the first place.

- Reduce distractions, such as other conversations taking place in the background or having the TV or radio on.

- Don't assume that every change is due to Parkinson disease. Be on the lookout for other issues and continue to assess the person's other health needs.

- If the person has had surgery, be sure the surgeon knows about the PD. Fasting and not taking Parkinson's medications before surgery can affect the person's mental state. Consult with the neurologist, who should consult with the surgeon as needed.

- Pick the best times of day for the person to take on tasks—when the effects of medication and the person's strength are at their highest.

- Write down how to operate TV, VCRs, and DVD players.

- If the person cooks, write down and follow recipes. Have the person check off the steps as they are done.

- Limit the person's use of alcohol.

- Put an alarm or a whistle in the bathroom in case the person needs to call for help.

Facial Exercises

Many individuals with PD perform face and mouth exercises to reduce the effects of muscle rigidity (tightness). From the following list, figure out which exercises are the most difficult for the person in your care to do. This will show the muscles that may need the most work.

Instructions are directed to the person with PD.

Start with 10 repetitions of each of the movements. If smiling is the exercise, smile as wide as possible and hold each smile for 5 to 10 seconds. Continue to breathe throughout the exercises. Practice in front of a mirror so that you can see the muscles work.

1. Smile – hold – relax – repeat.

2. Pucker your lips (in a kiss) – hold – relax – repeat.

3. Alternate puckering, then smiling.
   Pucker as tightly and smile as hard as you can. To increase the benefit of this exercise, knit your eyebrows together when you pucker, and raise the eyebrows when you smile.

4. Open your mouth and move the tip of your tongue all around the lips. The tongue should touch every part of the lips—bottom, top, both corners—slowly and not "darting" about.

5. Open your mouth and move the tongue around the gum line. Move your tongue over the back of top and bottom teeth, front of top and bottom teeth and each side of top and bottom teeth.

6. Open your mouth as wide as you can – hold – relax – repeat.

7. Say "KA" as loud and hard as you can and draw the sound out.

8. Say "PA"/"TA"/"KA" as loud and fast as you can.*

*Exercises adapted with permission from the National Parkinson Foundation. See *Parkinson Disease: Caring and Coping, Parkinson's Disease: Speaking Out, Parkinson Disease: Speech and Swallowing.* Patient education materials are available free of charge by calling the NPF or visiting their Web site.

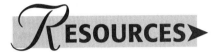

RESOURCES▸

For more information on the material presented in this chapter and free brochures on all topics related to Parkinson disease, contact:

American Parkinson Disease Association (APDA)
(800) 223-2732
www.apdaparkinson.org

European Parkinson's Disease Association (EPDA)
www.epda.eu.com

National Parkinson Foundation (NPF)
(800) 327-4545
www.parkinson.org

The following publications are available from the National Parkinson Foundation:
E-mail: mailbox@parkinson.org
Parkinson Disease: Caring and Coping
Parkinson's Disease: Speaking Out
Parkinson Disease: Speech and Swallowing (see Appendix B of this booklet for the anatomy of speech and communication)

American Association of Oral and Maxillofacial Surgeons
www.aaoms.org
Provides self-examination and oral cancer patient information on the Web site.

Meeting Life's Challenges
9042 Aspen Grove Lane
Madison, WI 53717
Fax (608) 824-0403
www.meetinglifeschallenges.com
E-mail: help@meetinglifeschallenges.com
Offers a guide called Dressing Tips and Clothing Resources for Making Life Easier, *by Shelley P. Schwartz, a guide to dressing for people with disabilities plus more than 100 resources for custome clothing.*

National Association for Continence (NAFC)
P.O. Box 8310
Spartanburg, SC 29305-8310
(800) 252-3337; (864) 579-7900; Fax: (864) 579-7902
www.nafc.org
NAFC is a leading source of education and support to the public about the diagnosis, treatments, and management alternatives for incontinence.

Publications

Speaking Effectively: A Strategic Guide for Speaking and Swallowing.
Vision Problems and Parkinson's Disease.
Both pamphlets available from the American Parkinson Disease Association by calling (800) 223-2732.
www.apdaparkinson.org
E-mail: apda@apdaparkinson.org

Mind, Mood, & Memory
National Parkinson Foundation
1501 N.W. 9th Avenue
Miami, FL 33136-1494
(800) 327-4545; (305) 243-6666
www.parkinson.org
E-mail: mailbox@parkinson.org

The following publication is available from the American Parkinson Disease Association:
Helping Your Partner: What Not to Do!

If you don't have home access to the Internet, ask your local library to help you locate any Web site.

Diet and Nutrition

Diet and Nutrition

Eat Well and Stay Active

It is important that a person with Parkinson disease stay healthy and active to help cope with PD as well as she or he possibly can. Try to serve a balanced diet to the person in your care. Make sure he or she gets regular exercise, even if it is only a short walk each day. Keep up enjoyable activities and social contacts with family and friends.

Healthy Eating

When someone has Parkinson disease or any chronic illness, it is important that she or he eats properly. The person will have more energy, his or her medication will work better, and he or she will feel more like exercising. A diet low in protein can benefit some people with Parkinson's disease, but attention must be paid to all nutritional needs.

A meal plan will help ensure that you are serving a balanced diet that includes fruit and vegetables, some high-protein foods, dairy products, and grains and cereals. Vitamin and mineral supplements are helpful for certain people. A dietician can help you plan a balanced diet for the person in your care.

It is also important for the person to take in plenty of fluids, especially water, and to stay away from caffeinated drinks (coffee, tea, soda) and alcohol.

A poor diet can result in the person's becoming weaker and at greater risk for infections. Check with the doctor before starting any special diets, especially for the person who has difficulty swallowing. Also, check with a doctor, pharmacist, or registered dietitian to know the effect of prescription medicines on nutritional needs.

> **NOTE** Do whatever possible to perk up the appetite. Food that is pleasing to look at will spark the appetite. Make sure the person's dentures fit correctly and that his or her glasses are the right prescription.

Principles of Good Nutrition

1. **Eat a variety of foods.**
   This includes food from each of the four food groups to ensure the right amounts of vitamins, minerals, carbohydrates, fats, and proteins.

2. **Eat less fat.**
   Eating a high-fat diet has been linked to heart disease. Fat can be lowered by eating more fish, poultry, and other lean meats. Drink low-fat milk and eat less ice cream, butter, and cheese.

3. **Eat more carbohydrates.**
   Eat more complex carbohydrates (starches, cereals, and breads), especially those high in fiber. They are a good source of energy, vitamins, and minerals.

4. **Maintain a reasonable weight.**
   The proper number of calories should be eaten to maintain ideal weight. The person with Parkinson disease is more likely to lose weight than to gain weight. Still, excess weight can affect the person's ability to get around.

5. **Avoid too much salt.**
   In Parkinson disease, blood pressure can often be too low. If this is the case and if there are no heart problems, then there is no need to avoid salt.

6. **Eat the right amount of fiber.**

   Fiber is the part of the plant cell that cannot be digested. Therefore, it cannot be absorbed by the bowel. Fiber is good for the health of the intestine and for regular bowel movements. The best sources of fiber are bran, fruits, vegetables, legumes, and whole-grain cereals. In Parkinson disease, fiber is important to prevent constipation. Fiber absorbs water (providing bulk), which then helps the bowel to empty itself.

Tip Antiparkinsonian drugs can cause nausea, vomiting, loss of appetite, and constipation. Nausea and loss of appetite usually occur when starting the drug and then lessen over time as people become used to the side effects. The person with continuing nausea and loss of appetite should be watched carefully for signs of poor nutrition.

NOTE Get a referral to a dietician to assess and set up a nutritional care plan. This plan should take into account the physical and social factors discussed above. It may require education of family members and referral to community supports, such as the Meals on Wheels program.

Diet and Parkinson Disease

Digestion

Parkinson disease can change the way the body digests food. People with PD can have problems taking in (absorbing) the nutrients they need from food. Several factors can result in weight loss. These include loss of taste, sense of smell, or appetite; feelings of nausea, difficulty swallowing, and increased energy needs. Most patients level off at a lower weight.

If the person in your care has any weight loss, notify the doctor or dietician. They can help you with a safe weight-gain plan if the person needs to put on weight.

Constipation

Constipation is another common problem that may affect a person with Parkinson disease. This is because of a slowing down of the muscle action that moves food through the gut. It is often a result of the PD itself and the medications used to treat it. Constipation can sometimes be managed with dietary changes, such as drinking plenty of water and increasing fiber. Foods such as whole-grain cereals, oat flakes, fruit (especially prunes), and vegetables with edible skins are a good source of fiber. However, if you are not used to eating whole-grain foods, increase the amount slowly over time.

NOTE If the person in your care is constipated, don't be embarrassed to discuss it with the doctor. Medication or referral to a specialist may be needed.

Management of Simple Constipation

1. Serve a balanced diet, including foods containing fiber.

2. Make sure the person gets plenty of rest and relaxation.

3. Have the person do moderate routine exercises.

4. Tell the person not to put off the urge to have a bowel movement.

5. Provide 6 to 8 glasses of water or noncaffeinated drinks per day.

6. Check with the health care provider to see if medications are causing the constipation.

7. Give the person a stool softener once or twice a day to manage simple constipation.

8. For more severe constipation, consult the health care provider.

Note that when used too often some laxatives can be toxic to the bowel. (📖 See *Activities of Daily Living*, pp. 165–168.)

NOTE Fluid intake of 6 to 8 glasses per day should be encouraged. Drinks that contain caffeine do not count, because they act as a diuretic, which removes fluids from the body. In Parkinson disease, fluid intake at this level is very important for reducing constipation.

Diet and PD Medications

Diet can also have an impact on the way PD medications work, particularly levodopa. Although levodopa preparations may be absorbed faster on an empty stomach, instructions usually advise taking the medication with food or milk if they upset the stomach.

- Meals can interfere with levodopa absorption because certain foods may delay levodopa's getting through the gut into the bloodstream and reaching the brain.

- Most people can take levodopa without having nausea and are able to take their medications before meals. For some people this may be 1 to 2 hours before eating. Others find it better to take their medication 30 minutes before eating.

- Some people find that avoiding high-protein foods during the day and eating them in the evening helps with mobility during the day. Red meat, poultry, fish, milk, cheese, eggs, seeds, and beans are all high in protein.

- Other individuals benefit from combining small amounts of protein with a high level of carbohydrates (for example, fruit, bread, cereal, pasta, and other grains) throughout the day. Eating fewer fatty foods may also help.

- Consult the doctor and/or a dietician to help set up a mealtime routine that suits the person's medications and daily activities.

Tip If it is difficult for the person in your care to swallow more than one pill, you may want to ask the doctor to decrease the number of pills or to give smaller pills.

A Special Diet for Parkinson Disease

Diet can alter how well levodopa works. The next section is only for those people taking levodopa who are having on-again-off-again problems with their mobility.

Diet and Levodopa

First, we must understand how levodopa works.

1. Levodopa leaves the blood rapidly, in about 60 to 90 minutes. Therefore, the blood levels of the drug fluctuate (go up and down). Anything that would delay levodopa's entering the bloodstream would also delay how much gets into the brain and how well the medication works.

2. Levodopa is not absorbed (taken in by the body) from the stomach, but from the small bowel. Therefore, anything that delays the emptying of the stomach contents into the small bowel can decrease absorption of the drug.

3. Proteins in the diet use the same method that levodopa does to get from the blood to the brain. Therefore, in some instances protein can slow down levodopa's ability to get to the brain.

4. Many dietary factors affect how rapidly the stomach empties its contents and therefore how quickly levodopa reaches the bloodstream and brain. Research shows that taking the drug with food can slow down absorption for some people.

Nutritional Guidelines for People with Parkinson Disease

PD slows gastric motility (stomach-emptying time). Chewing and swallowing are prolonged; stomach emptying is delayed, and food moves through the intestines more slowly than in someone who does not have PD. Nutrients are better absorbed when small amounts are eaten frequently rather than three large meals per day.

Most patients get more benefit from levodopa when taken on an empty stomach. A tablet, taken prior to eating (even 15 minutes is beneficial) *with 4–5 oz. nondairy fluid*, is "washed" from the stomach, through the pylorus valve, and into the small intestine, where absorption begins. Think of it as allowing the levodopa a "head start" on absorption before the food about to be eaten!

If levodopa causes nausea, a small cracker or bite of fruit can be taken with doses required between meals. Pretzels are an excellent choice because they require no refrigeration. Or, crystallized ginger can be nibbled to offset nausea. In extreme cases of levodopa-induced nausea, *motilium (Domperidone)* can be obtained from the U.K. or Canada.

A small percentage of people with PD benefit significantly from altering the amount or timing of protein intake to avoid interfering with levodopa absorption. These are typically patients who experience significant on/off motor fluctuations, and may take levodopa five or more times per day. To verify if protein is interfering with L-dopa absorption, experiment with a vegetarian diet for 3 days to determine whether levodopa function and motor benefit is significantly improved.

Weight maintenance is a problem for many people who have PD. Frequent, small meals can help maintain optimal weight. Liquid supplements can be useful. Sometimes patients are so diligent in limiting fat intake and worrying needlessly about protein restrictions, that they deprive themselves of much-needed calories.

Many dieticians recommend augmenting a well-balanced diet with a daily vitamin and mineral supplement as a nutritional "insurance policy." Do *not* choose a megadose formula. Always take supplements with food.

Tip

Our natural sense of thirst diminishes with age. Antiparkinson drugs also dry out the body. It is important to drink water "by the clock," not unlike one would schedule crucial medications. This allows better absorption of nutrients from foods as well as medications, and reduces the risk of dehydration.

Careful Food Preparation

People who are chronically ill or elderly are are more at risk from unsafe food, so be extra careful when preparing their meals.

- Wash your own hands and the hands of the person in your care with antibacterial soap before preparing or serving food.

- Dry hands with a paper towel.

- Use a solution of 1 teaspoon chlorine bleach per quart of water to kill germs in the sink and on kitchen counters.

- Air drying dishes is more sanitary than using a dish towel.

- Check expiration dates on labels, and throw out any food that is past the expiration date.

 If the water temperature is set too low, the dishwasher will not sterilize the dishes.

Nutrition Guidelines for Those Who Are Elderly

Be aware of any medical condition that would require limiting certain things, such as salt (in the case of congestive heart failure) or potassium (with kidney failure).

- Make tasty well-balanced meals that result in good bowel function and a normal flow of urine.

> *Tip* Ice in beverages may make swallowing and choking worse.

- Offer drinking water or liquids at mealtime to make chewing and swallowing easier.

- Avoid lard, bacon fat, coconut, and palm kernel oils, sweets, and highly seasoned foods.

- Serve fresh fruits and vegetables. They are good sources of fiber and vitamins A and C and they prevent constipation.

- Do not serve too much refined food. Refined foods are those that are processed, which removes nutrients and fiber and adds "bad" fats. Lack of fiber can lead to constipation.

- To improve poor appetites, use seasonings such as herbs, spices, lemon juice, peppers, garlic, and vinegar, especially if salt is restricted.

Boosting Calorie Intake

- Offer most of the food when the person is most hungry.

- Encourage the person to eat food with the fingers if it will increase how much the person eats.

- Add butter, whipped cream, or sour cream to foods.

- Add nuts, seeds, and wheat germ to breads, cereal, casseroles, and desserts.

- Add honey, jam, or sugar to bread, milk drinks, fruit, and yogurt desserts.

- Add mayo to salads and sandwiches.

Quick and Easy Snacks

Check first with the doctor to see if there should be a limit on sugar, salt, or potassium.

- cheese on crackers

- chocolate milk

- fruits, non-dairy "smoothies"

- granola cookies

- hard-boiled eggs

- puddings

- raisins, nuts, prunes

PREPARING FOOD

When preparing a meal for your family, put a small amount in the blender to make it easier for the person in your care to eat.

Therapeutic Diets

Keep the doctor informed about the diet you provide for the person in your care. A special diet may be prescribed to—

- improve or maintain a person's health

- increase (or decrease) the amount of fiber

- change to a soft diet

- remove or decrease certain foods

- change the number of calories

Preventing Dehydration

Dehydration is the absence or loss of fluids from the body. As a person ages, he or she feels less thirsty, so a special effort should be made to provide enough fluids. A person's fluid balance can be affected by medication, emotional stress, exercise, nourishment, general health, and the weather. In those who are elderly, dehydration can increase confusion and muscle weakness and cause nausea. Nausea will prevent the person from wanting to eat. The result is more dehydration.

Preventive measures include

- 6 to 8 cups of liquid every day (or an amount determined by the doctor)

- serving beverages at room temperature

- providing foods high in liquid (for example, watermelon)

- limiting caffeine and alcohol, which causes frequent urination and dehydration

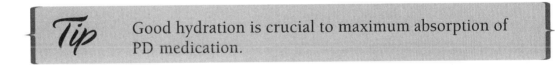

Tip   Good hydration is crucial to maximum absorption of PD medication.

Preventing Osteoporosis

Older people—especially women—often have osteoporosis. This condition occurs when minerals are lost from the bones. The bones then become weakened, break easily, and are slow to heal.

Osteoporosis can be prevented by

- getting enough vitamin D from sunshine a few times per week, and from fortified milk (not yogurt), fatty fish, or a vitamin supplement

- getting calcium from dairy foods, leafy vegetables such as kale and collards, broccoli, salmon, and sardines

- taking calcium citrate supplements

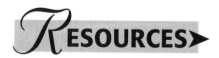

RESOURCES

For more information on the material presented in this chapter and free brochures on all topics related to Parkinson disease, contact:

American Parkinson Disease Association (APDA)
(800) 223-2732
www.apdaparkinson.org

European Parkinson's Disease Association (EPDA)
www.epda.eu.com

National Parkinson Foundation (NPF)
(800) 327-4545
www.parkinson.org

Publications

Eat Well, Stay Well with Parkinson's Disease
by Kathrynne Holden, MS, RD
Cook Well, Stay Well with Parkinson's Disease
by Kathrynne Holden, MS, RD
Eat Well *is a superb nutritional primer for people with PD,
whereas* Cook Well *offers an expanded recipe collection.
Available at www.nutritionucanlivewith.com*

Nutrition Matters
by Kathrynne Holden, MS RD
Available at no cost from the NPF.

Good Nutrition
Available from the American Parkinson Disease
Association.
Contains nutrition information and tasty recipes.

Dieticians

To get the number of a registered dietician in your area, check the yellow pages under "dietician." Be sure the dietician is registered or licensed. Or call the American Dietetic Association at (800) 877-1600, ext. 4898, and ask for the qualified dieticians in your area.

American Dietetic Association
(800) 366-1655
Call weekdays 10:00 a.m. to 5:00 p.m. EST to locate a registered dietitian in your area.

Area Agency on Aging or the Cooperative Extension Service
Your local office offers free counseling by a registered dietitian.

Dietary Specialties, Inc
P.O. Box 227
Rochester, NY 14601
(800) 544-0099; (716) 263-2787
Dietary Specialties offers a variety of low-protein foods. Call for a price list and order form.

Eldercare Locator
(800) 677-1116
Call to locate a senior nutrition center in your area.

Ener-G Food, Inc
5960 1st Avenue S
Seattle, WA 98124
(206) 767-6660
Ener-G Foods can provide low-protein recipes and foods.

F.D.A. Food Safety Information Hotline
(888) SAFE FOOD (723-3366)
www.fda.gov OR www.cfsan.fda.gov
Offers food safety and nutrition information in English and Spanish from specialists from 10:00 a.m. to 4:00 p.m. EST; provides recorded information 24 hours a day.

General Mills, Inc
P.O. Box 200
Minneapolis, MN 55440
(612) 540-2311
General Mills can provide information on the protein content of most foods.

Meals on Wheels
Can deliver nutritious meals to the home.

MyPyramid
www.mypyramid.gov
This replaces the old Food Guide Pyramid. It is a very interactive site to help people make health choices consistent with the 2005 Dietary Guidelines for Americans.

U.S.D.A. Meat and Poultry Hotline
(800) 535-4555
www.fsis.usda.gov
Provides recorded messages on food safety and preparation 24 hours a day, and specialists to answer specific questions from 10:00 a.m. to 4:00 p.m. EST.

If you don't have access to the Internet, ask your local library to help you locate any Web site.

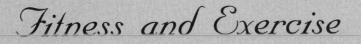

Fitness and Exercise

Fitness and Exercise

Exercise and PD

Some people don't exercise because they think it will be too difficult or that they don't have the time. Others simply do not understand how exercise can help them. Exercise is important for everyone. It is the basis for fitness, and it also helps fight the effects of aging and disease.

Exercise is even more important for a person with Parkinson disease. Regular exercise can help people with PD stay more flexible (able to bend), improve posture, and make overall movement (mobility) easier. Although medication has been the most effective treatment so far, a regular exercise program should always be part of managing PD. Exercise is one of the few treatments that is free, has no side effects, and can actually be enjoyable!

Though exercise is not a cure, it can help the person with PD stay ahead of the changes that will take place. It can help the person feel more in control of the condition.

Physical and Occupational Therapy

This book provides general information and suggestions about exercise for all people living with PD. A licensed physical therapist (PT) or occupational therapist (OT) can answer specific questions or problems you or the person in your care may have.

Physical and occupational therapists can do the following:

• Come up with an exercise program to meet the special needs of the person in your care.

- Assess and treat mobility problems (ability to get around) and walking problems.

- Assess and treat joint or muscle pain that affect the person's ability to perform activities of daily living.

- Help with poor balance or frequent falling.

- Teach caregivers proper body mechanics (position) and ways of assisting someone with PD.

- Refer the person to exercise programs in the community.

- Treat difficulties with the activities of daily living (ADL) such as eating, dressing, bathing, and handwriting.

- Teach the use of adaptive equipment (helping aids).

The doctor or other health care professional should be able to refer you to a therapist in your area. It is best to see a therapist who has special training or experience with PD. Visits to a physical or occupational therapist are usually covered by medical insurance with referral by a physician.

The Basics of Exercise

Good physical fitness is made up of three types of exercise: stretching, strengthening, and aerobics. Each is important by itself, but together they can help the person in your care remain active as long as possible. This will help the person deal better with PD and the changes it may bring.

A person should always stretch before exercise. This warms the muscles, helps prevent stiffness, and improves flexibility and balance. The person should work at his or her own pace, even if it seems very slow. Encourage the person in your care, even if the exercises seem difficult at first. Watch for signs of fatigue. Always cool down after exercise.

> **NOTE** Many of the suggestions in this section are geared to the person with PD. As caregiver, you can also take part in an exercise program. And you can offer support by helping the person practice and encouraging the person's efforts.

Stretching

Regular s-t-r-e-t-c-h-i-n-g is the first step, and it can be one of the most enjoyable. Stretching helps combat the muscle rigidity (stiffness) that comes with PD. It also helps muscles and joints stay flexible (able to bend). People who are more flexible have an easier time with everyday movement.

Stretching increases range of motion of joints and helps with good posture. It protects against muscle strains or sprains, improves circulation, and releases muscle tension.

Do's and Don'ts of Stretching

- DO stretch to the point of a gentle pull.

- DON'T stretch to the point of pain.

- DON'T bounce while stretching.

- DON'T hold the breath during a stretch. Breathe evenly in and out during each stretch.

- DON'T compare yourself to others.

Stretching can be done at any time. The person in your care can start the day by stretching before getting out of bed. Have the person stretch throughout the day, while watching television or riding in a car.

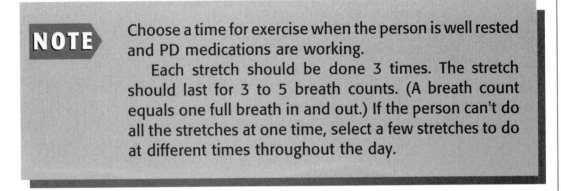

NOTE Choose a time for exercise when the person is well rested and PD medications are working.

Each stretch should be done 3 times. The stretch should last for 3 to 5 breath counts. (A breath count equals one full breath in and out.) If the person can't do all the stretches at one time, select a few stretches to do at different times throughout the day.

Deep Breathing

People with PD often take shallow breaths. Their lungs do not fill completely, which leads to tension and fatigue. (It can also affect the quality of speech.) Learning how to take full, deep breaths will expand the lungs, bring in more oxygen, and relax the person.

Practice breathing deeply:

1. Sit or lie down. Gently place the palms over the lower abdomen (stomach).

2. Take a full breath in through the nose (inhale), allowing the upper chest to expand. If the exercise is done correctly, the abdomen should lift.

3. Slowly breathe out (exhale) through the mouth. The exhale should last longer than the inhale.

4. Perform this exercise for 5 minutes a day, or at any time, to help feel relaxed.

Breathing Exercise

1. Stand tall with feet hip-width apart.

2. Cross arms over one another.

3. Take in a deep breath and begin lifting arms up and open.

4. Breathe out and lower hands to starting pose.

5. Perform for 5 deep breaths.

Strengthening

Strengthening is another important part of a PD exercise program. Strengthening certain muscles can help the person with PD stand up straighter. It can make certain tasks easier, such as getting up from a chair. These exercises also help to make bones stronger, so a person is less likely to get a fracture if he or she falls.

Let the person use hand-held weights if you have them. If there is access to a gym with weight machines, by all means go! However, strengthening exercises can be done in the privacy of the home. A person can build strength by using his or her own body weight as resistance. (Squats and being prone on the elbows are exercises that use a person's body weight as resistance.) The trick is to find out what kind of exercises work best for the person in your care.

Tools and Equipment

There are many tools available for building strong muscles and bones. Choose the one that best suits the person's situation and setting.

• small hand weights (available in sporting goods departments).

• wrist and ankle weights with Velcro® closures.

• elastic resistance bands such as TheraBands®.

Tip Many common household items can also be used for strengthening exercises.

- soup cans
- plastic shampoo or milk bottles filled with water or sand
- laundry detergent bottles

Aerobics

Aerobics (also known as conditioning exercise) includes any nonstop activity that uses the entire body. Aerobic exercises work the heart and lungs as well as muscles. Aerobic activities include—

- walking
- swimming
- water aerobics (aquatics)
- biking
- dancing

Some regular daily activities have an aerobic effect:

- household chores such as mopping or vacuuming
- walking the dog
- gardening and yard work

A program of regular aerobic exercise 3 or more times a week can—

- strengthen the heart and lungs
- improve energy and staying power
- reduce stress
- improve mood and fight depression
- help control high blood pressure, high cholesterol, and diabetes

Aerobics may also be done from a seated position. "Armchair aerobics" videos can be found at many sporting-goods stores or discount and department stores. **A person should get a doctor's approval before beginning any aerobic, or conditioning, program. This is especially important for those over 50 or those who have a history of cardiovascular (heart and blood vessel) disease.**

(See *Resources* for APDA's, *Be Active!*)

Balance

Reasons for Poor Balance

Balance problems are one of the main symptoms of PD. Balance problems increase the risk of falling, especially when combined with other symptoms of PD. These other symptoms include—

- slowness of movement (bradykinesia), which causes delayed reaction time
- stooped posture, which can cause the center of gravity to shift forward (the feeling of the feet having to "catch up" to the body)
- shuffling walk
- "freezing" in place
- falling backwards

Certain movements are likely to cause a person with PD to fall backward.

- opening a door by pulling it toward himself or herself
- backing up to sit down in a chair
- stepping backward to move away from something

Sometimes a person with PD will take quick, short steps forward and feels unable to stop. This tends to happen when the person—

- shuffles

- reaches too far ahead

- tries to fight through a "freeze"

- has dyskinesias (movements that the person cannot control)

Improving Balance

Balance exercises can help improve balance and decrease the chance of falling.

If the person in your care is having trouble with balance or is falling, ask the doctor or other health care professional to refer you to a physical therapist. The therapist can suggest exercises, equipment, and methods to improve balance and reduce falls.

Falls

Preventing Falls

With PD, a person now must think about many things that he or she was able to do easily before. These tips are intended for the person with PD to reduce falls:

1. Try not to move too quickly. **Think** about what you are doing.

2. When walking, the foot should land with the heel striking down first.

3. **DO NOT** pivot the body over the feet when turning. Instead, try making a "U-turn" while walking.

4. When standing in place and ready to turn, make sure the feet and the body move together.

5. Never lean too far forward. If you must lean forward

- widen your stance and place one foot ahead of the other;

- stand directly in front of what you are reaching for;

- place one hand on the counter, wall, or other steady object while you reach with your other hand.

6. The moment you begin to shuffle or freeze, try to come to a complete stop. Take a breath and start again, focusing on that first step and striking down heel first.

7. Do not carry too many things while you are walking. It only makes your task more difficult.

8. Avoid walking backwards. Instead, try—

   - stepping sideways

   - taking large marching steps to turn and then walking forward

   - when returning to sit, turn all the way around and make sure that the backs of both legs are touching the chair. Reach back with both arms to lower yourself slowly. NEVER reach forward for the chair first and then turn to sit.

When There Are Falls

People who fall frequently should be enrolled in an emergency signaling system. Protective equipment such as knee and elbow pads can help prevent injuries.

A physical or occupational therapist can teach you and the person in your care the best techniques for getting up from the floor after a fall.

(Check local programs in your community on fall-prevention classes.)

Posture

PD can cause many changes in the body. One of the most noticeable changes is the posture. Changes in posture can include the following:

- a forward head position

- rounding of the shoulders and upper back

- a forward trunk position with increased bending of the hips and knees

Exercise and proper body positions can help limit or correct these changes. There are other reasons for poor posture, including—

- sitting on the couch watching TV

- leaning over to work on the computer

- driving or riding in the car

- looking down while reading, or propping one's head against the headboard while reading.

Maintaining Good Posture

Fortunately, there are some easy ways to break these bad habits.

The following tips are helpful for anyone wishing to maintain good posture. **They are *extremely* important for persons with PD:**

Sitting

1. Avoid sitting in chairs without back support or armrests.

2. Avoid recliners. They cause rounding of the neck, shoulders, and head, and also tightness in the hips.

3. Avoid low, soft couches and chairs.

4. The height of the chair should allow for the hips and knees to be level with one another.

5. Keep the chin parallel to the floor.

6. Avoid crossing the legs.

7. Keep the head, shoulders, and hips in line with one another. Sit so that your back is fully in contact with the chair back and seat.

8. A lumbar roll along the low back will help a person sit tall (especially on long car rides, plane rides, and in the theater).

9. Computer screens and TVs should be at eye level to cut down on neck and eyestrain.

10. Use a bookstand or rest your elbows on a pillow or a table when reading. Look directly ahead at the pages. When reading in bed, the entire back should rest along the headboard.

11. **DO NOT** sit for long periods at a time. Get up and move around after about 20 or 30 minutes.

Standing and Walking

1. Keep chin parallel to the floor.

2. **DO NOT** look straight down while walking.

3. Keep a broad base of support by keeping feet at shoulder width.

4. Keep the shoulders rolled back, and head and chest up.

Lying Down

1. Avoid using too many pillows, or too thin a pillow, under the head.

2. The best postures for sleeping are lying on the back with a soft pillow under the knees; or lying on the side with a soft pillow between the knees.

Other Hints for Good Posture

1. Perform frequent neck and shoulder stretches to relieve muscle tension.

2. Maintain eye contact during conversation. This holds the head erect.

3. Avoid sleeping in a chair. Lie down to nap with the head and neck supported.

4. Practice these techniques every day.

5. Place written reminders on the bathroom mirror, computer screen, dashboard, and television. "Stand tall. Shoulders back. Sit straight. Chin up."

6. See a physical or occupational therapist for specific posture exercises.

Complementary Therapies

Aquatic Exercises

Water therapy is a time-tested form of healing. It is also a safe exercise for people with PD because there is no danger of falling. Floating in the water allows for easy movement and little strain on joints and muscles. Look to see if your community has a heated pool that offers an exercise program. (See **Resources** for APDA's, *Aquatic Exercise for PD.*)

Massage Therapy

Massage therapy increases circulation (blood flow), reduces muscle tension, and helps a person relax. It can be very useful to the person with PD who experiences problems with rigidity (stiffness). Massage should be part of an overall fitness program that includes regular movement and exercise.

Select a massage therapist who is certified by the American Massage Therapy Association. Talk to the therapist about methods. The person with PD should provide feedback during the massage in the event of any discomfort. Self-massage and massage provided by the caregiver are also possible. Using items such as wooden rollers or hand-held electric massagers will allow you or the person in your care to apply gentle pressure to tight areas of the body. These items can be purchased at most drug or department stores. Massage services are often not covered by health insurance.

Tai Chi

Tai chi is a slow, flowing form of ancient Chinese exercise. It aids in flexibility, balance, and relaxation. Many people with Parkinson's disease have been helped by doing tai chi. Several forms of tai chi can be done by anyone regardless of age or physical condition. Classes are often offered at fitness centers, senior centers, and community recreation centers. Speak with the instructor to learn if the type of tai chi he or she teaches is best for the person in your care. Tai chi programs are also available on videotape at a variety of retail stores.

Yoga

Yoga is a form of exercise that can be very helpful for persons with PD. It increases flexibility, relaxation, and awareness of breathing and posture. Yoga also can reduce stress. Yoga is self-paced, which means that people can do the poses in their own way and hold the pose for as long as they are comfortable. Yoga can even be done in a chair. It is important to contact the instructor prior to beginning a class. Generally, a beginner class or a class for those with special needs is a good place to start for those with PD.

> *Tip*
> If the person in your care has significant balance impairment, Tai Chi and yoga moves from a chair may be necessary.

Pet Therapy

"Lap" pets, such as dogs and cats, can provide great joy in the lives of their human friends. Having animals in the home improves the mental and emotional health of their owners. It also provides movement and exercise. According to research, pets can—

- lower blood pressure and heart rate

- improve mobility and flexibility (through stroking, grooming, and walking the pet)

- satisfy the human need for touch and caring for another

Independence Dogs

People with mobility impairments can gain independence through the help of specially trained dogs. These dogs are trained by organizations such as Independence Inc., a non-profit school, to provide physical, psychological, and therapeutic support for their human partners.

Wheelchair dogs are taught to pull their partners up ramps and to provide support for their partners as they transfer to and from the wheelchair. These dogs can also help a partner get back into the chair after a fall. The dogs also help by opening doors and carrying things in special backpacks.

Walker dogs are trained to help people who cannot walk without the aid of mobility devices. By leaning on a dog wearing a specially designed harness, the person can get up and down stairs and into and out of cars. These dogs also retrieve dropped articles, can get a cordless telephone, as well as carry items in a backpack, and open doors.

Creative Expression

Creative expression can provide movement and physical activity. Painting on an easel with large, strong strokes stretches the arms and shoulders. "Conducting" the music of a favorite symphony or opera has shown to have a strengthening and aerobic benefit. Singing alone or in a choral group promotes the deep breathing needed for louder speech. Encourage the person in your care to seek creative outlets that fit their talents and abilities.

Exercises and the Daily Routine

A good exercise regimen can help a person with PD maintain mobility.

Persons with advancing Parkinson symptoms may not be able to follow some exercise programs due to changes in their physical or thinking abilities. It may be better to fit exercises and stretching into the daily routine:

- Find a simple activity that the person with PD enjoys, such as walking, gardening, housekeeping, or swimming. As caregiver, you can try to make some of these activities part of the daily routine.

- Sitting and reaching in different directions can stretch the arms and trunk.

- Household chores such as folding laundry, dusting, wiping dishes, or helping with food preparation provide gentle exercise.

- Simple games like balloon volleyball, playing catch with a large, soft ball or blowing soap bubbles are an enjoyable way to get exercise.

- Music creates movement such as marching or dancing. If balance is a problem, try chair dancing. "Conducting" to the beat of up-tempo music provides upper body exercise and good emotional therapy!

- Perform a few extra arm and leg motions during dressing tasks.

A physical therapist can suggest exercises and stretches that will suit the person with PD. Therapists can also provide ways to improve walking and balance.

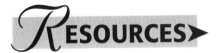

RESOURCES

For more information on the material presented in this chapter, and free brochures on all topics related to Parkinson disease, contact:

American Parkinson Disease Association (APDA)
(800) 223-2732
www.apdaparkinson.org

European Parkinson's Disease Association (EPDA)
www.epda.eu.com

National Parkinson Foundation (NPF)
(800) 327-4545
www.parkinson.org

Canine Partners for Life
#130D, R.D. #2
Cochranville, PA 19330
(610) 869-4902

Fidos for Freedom, Inc.
P.O. Box 5508
Laurel, MD 20726
(410) 880-4178

Independence Dogs Inc.
146 State Line Road
Chadds Ford, PA 19317

K-9 Service Dogs of NJ
144 N. Beverwyck Road, Suite 145
Lake Hiawatha, NJ 07034
(201) 335-7144

The following booklets are available from the American Parkinson Disease Association.

Be Active! A Suggested Exercise Program for People with Parkinson's Disease

Aquatic Exercise for PD

Body Mechanics—Positioning, Moving, and Transfers

Body Mechanics—Positioning, Moving, and Transfers

Body Mechanics for the Caregiver

Body mechanics involves standing and moving one's body to prevent injury, avoid fatigue, and make the best use of strength. When you learn how to control and balance your own body, you can safely control and move another person. Back injuries to nursing home aides are common, so when doing any lifting be sure to use proper body mechanics.

General Rules

- Never lift more than you can comfortably handle.

- Create a base of support by standing with your feet 8 to 12″ (shoulder width) apart with one foot a half step ahead of the other.

Proper foot position. ▶

- DO NOT let your back do the heavy work—USE YOUR LEGS. (The back muscles are not your strongest muscles.)

- If the bed is low, put one foot on a footstool. This relieves pressure on your lower back.

- Consider using a support belt for your back.

Helpful Caregiver Advice for Moving a Person

These pointers are for the *caregiver* only. Be sure to see the following pages for the steps for a specific move or transfer.

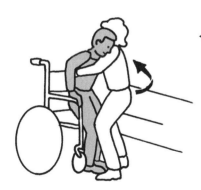

◀**1**
- Tell the person what you are going to do.
- Before starting a move, count with the person, "1-2-3."

◀**2**
- To feel in control, get close to the person you are lifting.
- While lifting, keep your back in a neutral position (arched normally, not stiff), knees bent, weight balanced on both feet. Tighten your stomach and back muscles to maintain a correct support position.
- Use your arms to support the person.
- Again, *let your legs do the lifting.*

◀**3**
- Pivot (turn on one foot) instead of twisting your body.
- Breathe deeply.
- Keep your shoulders relaxed.
- When a lot of assistance is needed with transfers, tie a strong belt or a transfer belt around the person's waist and hold it as you complete the transfer.

NOTE To encourage independence, let the person make a few attempts at helping. It's okay for him to stand part-way up and sit back down.

Preventing Back and Neck Injuries

To prevent injuries to yourself, get plenty of rest and follow a healthful lifestyle that includes

- good nutrition
- physical fitness
- good body mechanics
- a program for managing stress

Common Treatments for Caregiver Back Pain

If you *do* experience back pain:

- Apply a cold ice pack to the injured area for 10 minutes every hour (you can use a bag of frozen vegetables).
- Get short rest periods in a comfortable position.
- Stand with your feet shoulder width apart. With hands on hips, bend backwards. Do 3 to 5 repetitions several times a day.
- Take short, frequent walks on a level surface.
- Avoid sitting for long periods. Sitting is one of the worst healing positions.

Tip **PREVENTING BACK INJURIES**
Having the person grab a trapeze to help with the move is easiest and safest for your back. (📖 See p. 85.)

As the caregiver, you should seek training from a physical therapist to provide this type of care to reduce the risk of injury to yourself or the person in your care. The therapist will correct any mistakes you make and can take into account special problems. To determine the best procedure for you to use, the therapist will consider the physical condition of the person you care for and the furniture and room arrangements in the home.

Moving a Person

Positioning a Person in Bed

- Place a small pillow under the person's head, keeping his spine neutral.

1 ▶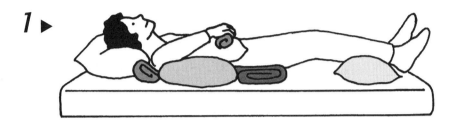

- Place a small pillow lengthwise under the calf of the weak leg, let the heel hang off the end of the pillow to prevent pressure, and loosen the top sheet to avoid pressure on the toes.

2 ▶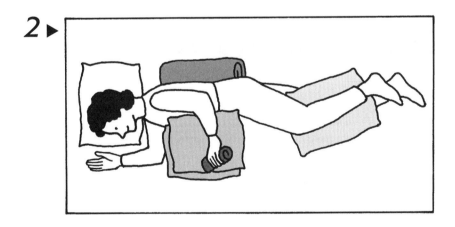

- Fold a bath towel under the hip of the person's weak side.
- Place the weak arm and elbow on a pillow higher than the heart.

Positioning a Person on His or Her Strong Side

1. Place a small pillow under the person's head.

2. Keep the person's head in alignment with the spine.

3. Place a rolled pillow at the back to prevent rolling.

4. Place a pillow in front to keep the arm the same height as the shoulder joint.

5. Place a medium pillow lengthwise between the knees, legs, and ankles. (The person's knees may be bent slightly.)

Positioning a Person on His or Her Weak Side

1. Use the same positioning as described above.

2. Change the person's position frequently because he may not be aware of pressure, pain, or skin irritation.

Moving a person in bed can injure the person in care or the caregiver if certain basic rules are not followed:

• Never grab or pull the person's arm or leg.

• If the medical condition allows, raise the foot of the bed slightly to prevent the person from sliding down.

• If moving him is difficult, get him out of bed and back in the wheelchair and start over by putting him in bed closer to the headboard.

Moving a Person Up in Bed

1. Tell the person what you are going to do.

2. Lower the head of the bed to a flat position and remove the pillow—never try to move the person "uphill."

3. If possible, raise the bed and **lock the wheels**.

4. Tell the person to bend the knees and brace the feet firmly against the mattress to help push.

5. Stand at the side of the bed and place one hand behind the person's back and the other underneath the buttocks.

6. Bend your knees and keep your back in a neutral position.

7. Count "1-2-3" and have the person push with the feet and pull with the hands toward the head of the bed.

8. Replace the pillow under his head.

 NOTE A draw sheet—a sheet folded several times and positioned under the person to be moved in bed—prevents irritation to the skin. The sheet should be positioned from the shoulders to just below the knees.

Moving the Person to One Side of the Bed on His or Her Back

1.
- Place your feet 8 to 12″ apart, knees bent, back in a neutral position.
- Slide your arms under the person's back to his far shoulder blade. (Bend your knees and hips to lower yourself to the person's level.)
- Slide the person's shoulders toward you by rocking your weight to your back foot.

2.
- Use the same procedure at the person's buttocks and feet.
- Always keep your knees bent and your back in a neutral position.

1 ▾   **2 ▾**

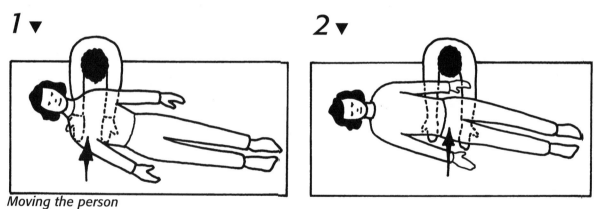

Moving the person

Rolling Technique

1. Move the person to one side of the bed as in the above procedure.

2. Bend the person's knees.

3. Hold the person at his hip and shoulder blade on the far side of the body.

4. Roll the person toward you to make sure he does not fall off the bed.

Raising the Person's Head and Shoulders

1. If possible, ask the person to lift the head and dig both elbows into the bed to support the body.

2. Face the head of the bed, feet 8 to 12" apart, knees bent, back in neutral.

3. Help the person lift his shoulders by placing your hands and forearms under the pillow and the person's shoulder blades.

4. Use bent knees, back in neutral, and locked arms to assist the lift.

5. Adjust the pillow.

Helping a Person Sit Up

1. Tell the person what you are going to do.

2. Bend the person's knees.

3. Roll her on her side to face you.

4. Reach one arm under her shoulder blade.

5. Place the other arm in back of the knees.

6. Position your feet 8 to 12" apart with your center of gravity close to the bed and person.

7. Keep your back in a neutral position.

8. Count "1-2-3" and shift your weight to your back leg.

9. Shift the person's legs over the edge of the bed while pulling her shoulders to a sitting position.

10. Remain in front of her until she is stabilized.

Rest and Sleeping

It is common for a person with PD to have trouble turning over or getting in and out of bed. These tips may help:

- If the person is having trouble getting in and out of bed or turning over in bed, talk to the health care provider. Medication may have to be adjusted.

- A satin sheet or piece of satin material tucked across the middle of the bed can make it easier for the person to turn over.

- Flannel sheets and heavy blankets can make it more difficult to turn over.

- Make sure the path from the bed to the bathroom is well lighted. Use a nightlight or leave open a closet door with the light left on.

- Keep the bedroom floor clear of things that could cause tripping and falling. Don't leave shoes, books, or papers on the floor.

Getting Up from Bed and Lying Down

To help the person in your care get up from bed, explain and repeat the following steps:

1. Bend knees up. Place feet flat on bed.

2. Turn onto side. Reach arm across body to assist rolling.

3. Move feet off edge of bed.

4. Use arms to push self into sitting position. (A half-side rail or chair fastened to the side of the bed may help.)

To help the person lie down in bed, explain and repeat the following steps:

1. Sit on edge of bed.

2. Lift legs into bed (one at a time may be easier).

3. Lie down with head on pillow.

4. Slide legs into center of bed (moving one leg at a time may be easier.)

Helping Someone Get Into Bed

1. Have the person approach the bed as if he were going to sit in a chair. He should feel the mattress behind both legs.

2. Have the person slowly lower himself to a seated position on the bed, using his arms to control the lowering.

3. Tell him to lean on his forearm while allowing his trunk to lean down to the side.

4. As the trunk goes down, the legs will want to go up, like a seesaw.

5. Do not have the person place his knees up on the mattress first. In other words, he shouldn't "crawl" into bed.

Helping Someone Get Out of Bed

1. Have the person bend the knees up, feet flat on the bed.

2. Tell him to roll onto his side toward the edge of the bed by letting his knees fall to that side. Tell him to turn his head and look in the direction he is rolling.

3. Have him lower his feet from the bed and push with his arms into a sitting position.

4. A straight-back chair anchored at the side of the bed or a bed rail can help the person roll more easily.

Transfers

Transferring a person in and out of bed is an important caregiver activity. It can be done fairly easily if these instructions are followed. Use the same procedure for all transfers so that a routine is set up.

Helping a Person Stand

Help only as much as needed but guard the person from falling.

1. Have her sit on the edge of the chair or bed. Let her rest a moment if she feels lightheaded.

2. Instruct the person to push off with the hands from the bed or chair armrests.

3. Position your knee between the person's knees.

4. Face the person and support the weak knee against one or both of your knees as needed.

5. Put your arms around the person's waist or use a transfer belt.

6. Keep your back in a neutral position.

7. At the count of "1-2-3," instruct the person to stand up while pulling the person toward you and pushing your knees into the person's knee if needed.

8. Once she is upright, have her keep the knee locked straight.

9. Support and balance her as needed.

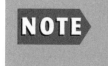

NOTE If during a transfer you start to "lose" the person, do not try to hold the person up. Instead, lower the person to the floor.

Helping a Person Sit

1. Reverse the process described in Helping a Person Stand.

2. Direct the person to feel for the chair or bed with the back of the legs.

3. Direct the person to reach back with both hands to the bed or chair armrests and slowly sit.

Transferring from Bed to Wheelchair With a Transfer Belt

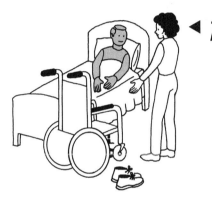

◀ **1** • Place the wheelchair at a 45° angle to the bed so that the person will be transferring to his or her stronger side.

  • **Lock the wheels** of the chair and the bed.

  • Tell the person what you are going to do.

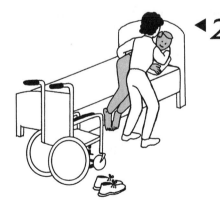

◀ **2** • Put on his shoes while he is still lying down if he is weak or unstable.

  • Bring him to a sitting position with his legs over the edge of the bed.

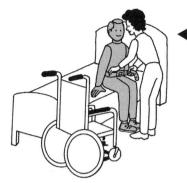

◀ **3** • Let him rest a moment if he feels lightheaded.

• Use a **transfer belt** for a person needing a lot of support.

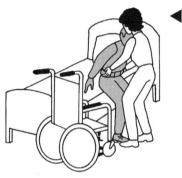

◀ **4** • Bring the person to a standing position as described on p. 236.

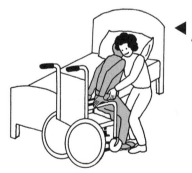

◀ **5** • Have him reach for the chair arm and pivot. A very fast pivot may frighten the person—or cause you to lose knee control and fall with a person who is totally dependent.

• Support him with your arms and knees as needed.

• Adjust him comfortably in the chair.

NOTE ▶ If the person starts to slide off the edge of the bed before or after the transfer, lay his upper torso across the bed to prevent him from falling to the floor.

Transferring from Wheelchair to Bed

1. Reverse the process described in Transfer from Bed to Wheelchair.

2. Place the chair at a 45° angle to the bed so the person is on his stronger side. **Lock the wheels**.

3. Get into a position to provide a good base of support; use good body mechanics.

4. Have the person stand, reach for the bed, and pivot.

5. Support and guide him as needed.

6. Adjust the person in bed with pillows.

Transferring from Bed to Wheelchair Without a Transfer Belt

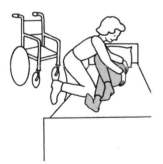

- Place the wheelchair at a 45° angle to the bed so that the person will be transferring to his stronger side.

- **Lock the wheels** of the chair (you can use a wheel block) and the wheels of the bed.

- Tell the person what you are going to do.

- Bring him to a sitting position with his legs over the edge of the bed following steps a, b, c, and d.

1a ▲

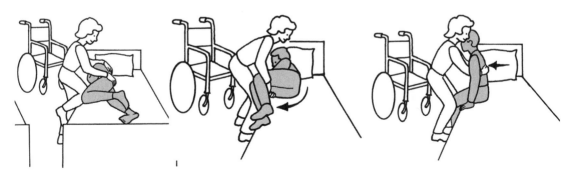

1b ▲   *1c* ▲   *1d* ▲

- Let him rest a moment if he feels lightheaded.
- Put his shoes on.

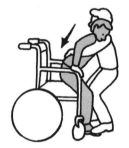

◀ **2** • Put your arms around his chest and clasp your hands behind his back.
- Support the leg that is farther from the wheelchair between your legs.

◀ **3** • Lean back, shift your leg, and lift.
- Pivot toward the chair.

◀ **4** • Bend your knees and let the person bend toward you.
- Lower the person into the wheelchair.
- Adjust him comfortably in the chair.

NOTE ▶ As the person becomes stronger, you can provide less assistance. However, use the same body positioning to support the person's weaker side.

Transferring from a Wheelchair to a Car

Be sure the car is parked on a level surface without cracks or potholes.

1 • Open the passenger door as far as possible.

• Move the left side of the wheelchair as close to the car seat as possible.

• **Lock the chair's wheels**.

• Move both footrests out of the way.

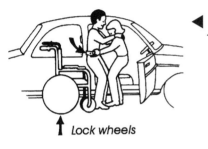

↑ *Lock wheels*

◀*2* • Position yourself facing the person.

• Tell the person what you are going to do.

• Bending your knees and hips, lower yourself to his level.

• By grasping the transfer belt around his waist help him stand while straightening your hips and knees.

• If his legs are weak, brace his knees with your knees.

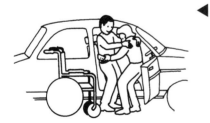

◀*3* • While he is standing, turn him so he can be eased down to sit on the car seat. GUIDE HIS HEAD so it is not bumped.

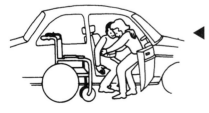

◀*4* • Lift his legs into the car by putting your hands under his knees.

• Move him to face the front.

• Put on his seat belt.

• Close door carefully.

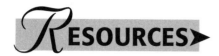

RESOURCES

American Academy of Orthopaedic Surgeons
6300 N. River Road
Rosemont, IL 60018
(800) 346-AAOS (800-346-2267)
www.aaos.org
Offers a free booklet Lift It Safe *on lifting procedures for home-based caregivers.*

If you don't have access to the Internet, ask your local library to help you locate a Web site.

Emergencies

Emergencies

*E*mergency situations are common with the elderly because of their chronic illnesses and problems resulting from falls. Many injuries can be avoided through preventive measures (see **Preparing the Home**, p. 59). But when a crisis does occur, use common sense, stay calm, and realize that you can help.

NOTE Make sure 911 is posted on your phone or ideally is on speed-dial. Keep written directions near the phone for how to get to your house. If you have a speakerphone, use the speaker when talking to the dispatcher. This way, you can follow the dispatcher's instructions while attending to the emergency.

When to Call for an Ambulance

A trip to the ER is useful for evaluating many things, but not Parkinson disease. You should go to the ER if you think the person in your care has an infection that is making the PD worse. Go to the ER if the person has fallen and you are worried about a broken bone or blood clot on the brain. **But never go to the ER just because the person's PD has gotten worse.**

The neurologist on your health care team has been working to treat and control the person's PD. ER doctors do not know about PD, and a 30-minute visit could undo whatever progress the neurologist has made. The person could be diagnosed with a stroke, have to undergo needless testing or treatments, and possibly wind up spending days in the hospital needlessly. (See *Resources for APDA's, Why Parkinson Disease Patients Should Not Go to the Emergency Room.*)

Do call for an ambulance if a person—

- becomes unconscious
- has chest pain or pressure
- has trouble breathing
- has no signs of breathing (no movement or response to touch or voice)
- is bleeding severely
- is vomiting blood or is bleeding from the rectum
- has fallen and may have broken bones
- has had a seizure
- has a severe headache and slurred speech
- has pressure or severe pain in the abdomen that does not go away

OR

- if moving the person could cause further injury
- if traffic or distance would cause a life-threatening delay in getting to the hospital
- if the person is too heavy for you to lift or help

Ambulance service is costly and may not be covered by insurance. Use it only when you believe there is an emergency. In an emergency:

Step 1: Call 911.
Step 2: Care for the victim.

Also call 911 for emergencies involving fire, explosion, poisonous gas, downed electrical wires, or other life-threatening situations.

> **NOTE** If the person in your care has a signed Do Not Resuscitate (DNR) order, have it available to show the paramedics. Otherwise, they are required to begin reviving the person. The DNR must go with the person if he is taken to the hospital and *must* be with the person at all times.

In the Emergency Room

Be sure you understand the instructions for care before leaving the emergency room. Call the person's personal doctor as soon as possible and let him or her know about the emergency room care.

Bring to the emergency room—

- insurance policy numbers
- a list of medical problems
- a list of medications currently being taken
- the personal physician's name and phone number
- the name and number of a relative or friend of the person in your care

We strongly suggest that you take a course in CPR from your local American Red Cross, hospital, or other agency.

Choking (Adult)

Prevention (See *Eating*, p. 175 and *Speech and Swallowing*, p. 178)

- Avoid serving excessive alcohol.
- Make sure the person in your care has a good set of dentures to chew food properly.
- Cut the food into small pieces.
- For a person who has had a stroke, use thickening powder in liquids.
- Do not encourage the person to talk while eating.
- Do not make the person laugh while eating.
- Learn the Heimlich maneuver in CPR class.

If the Adult Is Choking—Heimlich Maneuver

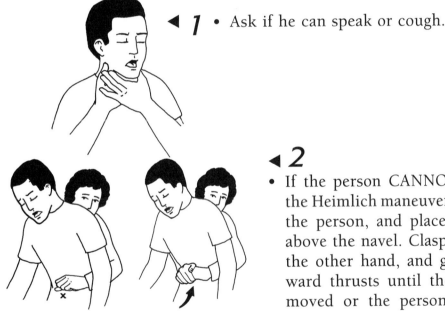

◄ **1** • Ask if he can speak or cough.

◄ **2**

• If the person CANNOT SPEAK, use the Heimlich maneuver: Stand behind the person, and place your fist just above the navel. Clasp your fist with the other hand, and give quick, upward thrusts until the object is removed or the person becomes unconscious.

3 If the person becomes *unconscious*, lower the person to the floor onto his back.

4 Call 911.

5 Tilt the head back and lift the chin to open the airway. Sweep the mouth with your fingers to remove any objects.

6 Place your mouth over the victim's mouth and try to give 2 breaths. Reposition the head if necessary and try to give 2 more breaths.

7 Repeat steps 5 and 6 until help arrives.

OR

- If breathing starts, place the person on his side in the **RECOVERY POSITION** (see illustration).

▶ *Placing a person in the Recovery Position.*

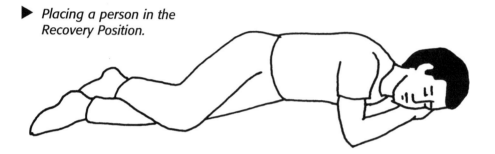

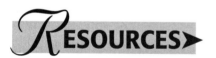

For more information on the material presented in this chapter, and free brochures on all topics related to Parkinson disease, contact:

American Parkinson Disease Association (APDA)
(800) 223-2732
www.apdaparkinson.org

European Parkinson's Disease Association (EPDA)
www.epda.eu.com

National Parkinson Foundation (NPF)
(800) 327-4545
www.parkinson.org

The following publication is available from the American Parkinson Disease Association:
Why Parkinson's Disease Patients Should Not Go to the Emergency Room

American Heart Association
National Center
7272 Greenville Avenue
Dallas, TX 75231
(800) AHA-USA1
www.AmericanHeart.org

American Red Cross
2025 E. Street N.W.
Washington, DC 20006
(202) 303-4498
www.RedCross.org

British Red Cross
UK Office
44 Moorfields
London EC2Y 9AL
Phone: 0870170 7000
www.redcross.org/uk

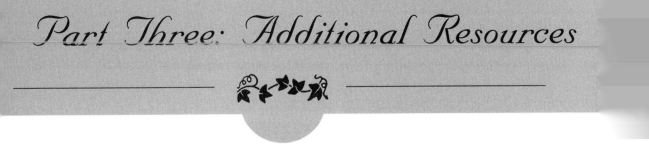

Part Three: Additional Resources

United States Parkinson Disease Organizations

American Parkinson Disease Association
125 Parkinson Avenue
Staten Island, NY 10305
(800)223-2732
(718) 981-8001
E-Mail: apda@apdaparkinson.org
www.parkinson.org
A comprehensive network of information and referral centers in the U.S. Excellent research funding and patient services in most states.

Michael J. Fox Foundation for Parkinson's Research
Grand Central Station
PO Box 4777
New York, NY 10163
www.michaeljfox.org
Raises money for research; excellent medical advisory board.

National Parkinson Foundation
1501 N.W. 9th Avenue / Bob Hope Road
Miami, FL 33136-1494
(305) 243-6666
(800) 327-4545
Fax: (305) 243-5595
www.parkinson.org
Funds Centers of Excellence, Care Centers, and Outreach Centers for research, care, and quality of life for patients and caregivers worldwide. For a listing of Centers, Chapters, support groups, and physicians, visit www.parkinson. org and click on the tab called "Find Resources."

The Parkinson Alliance
211 College Road East
3rd Floor
Princeton, NJ 08520
(609) 688-0870
Toll Free: (800) 579-8440
Fax: (609) 688-0875
E-mail: admin@parkinsonalliance.net
All funds go to research; umbrella organization sponsoring annual Unity Walk NYC and Team Parkinson at the Los Angles Marathon.

Parkinson's Action Network
300 North Lee Street
Alexandria, VA 22314
(703) 518-8877/ (800) 850-4726
Fax: (703) 518-0673
E-mail: info@parkinsonsaction.org
Coordinates political action efforts for PD in the U.S.

Parkinson's Disease Foundation
1359 Broadway, Suite 1509
New York, NY 10018
(800)457-6676
info@pdf.org
www.pdf.org
Research funding and educational support for families and health professionals: associated with Columbia University in NYC.

WE MOVE
204 West 84th Street
New York, NY 10024
www.wemove.org or www.mdvu.org (Movement Disorders Virtual University)
Worldwide education and awareness for movement disorders. The Internet's most comprehensive resource for movement-disorder information and the hub of movement-disorder activities on the Web. Outstanding scholarly references for lay people and health professionals. Strong links to other organizations links to PD clinical trial information.

Young Parkinson's Information & Referral Center

2100 Pfingsten Road
Glenview, IL 60026
(800)223-9776
www.youngparkinsons.org
E-Mail: info@youngparkinsons.org
Helps those with young-onset PD deal with issues, questions, and concerns, such as relationship issues with spouses, parents, children; accurate and age-specific medical information from the experts; common psychological/emotional issues; career and financial planning for the long term; news on current medical research; contact with other young people with PD.

Worldwide Parkinson Disease Associations*

European Parkinson's Disease Association

4 Golding Road
Sevenoaks
Kent, UK TN13 3NJ
E-mail: lizzie@epda.eu.com
www.epda.eu.com
Provides excellent patient information and works to promote international understanding of Parkinson disease, enabling people living with PD and their families to draw on best caring practice worldwide, to access the latest medical and surgical advice and thus make informed choices to achieve the best quality of life possible. Links to international PD organizations.

*Because of limited space we cannot list all organizations. Exclusion does not mean they are not valuable. Please visit www.epda.eu.com (European Parkinson's Disease Association) or www.wpda.org (World Parkinson Disease Association) for links to individual countries.

World Parkinson Disease Association
Via Zuretti 35, 20125 Milano, Italy
(+39) 02 6671 3111
Fax: (+39) 02 6705 283
E-mail: info@wpda.org

AUSTRALIA
Parkinson's Australia, Inc.
c/o Parkinson's New South Wales
Concord RG Hospital, Building 64
Hospital Road, Concord NSW 2139
(+61) 02 9767 7881
Fax: (+61) 02 9767 7882
Toll Free 1 (800) 644 189 (Inside Australia)
www.parkinsons.org.au
Email: Parkinsonsaus@bigpond.com

AUSTRALIAN CAPITAL TERRITORY
Parkinson's Disease Society of the ACT Inc
PO Box 717, Mawson, Australian Capital Territory 2607
(+61) 02 6290 1984
Fax: (+61) 02 6286 4475
Freecall: 1800 644 189 (Inside Australia)

AUSTRALIA QUEENSLAND
Parkinson's Queensland Inc.
PO Box 460, 26 Stoneham Street, Stones Corner 4120,
Queensland
(+61) 07 3397 7555
Fax: (+61) 07 3397 1755
E-mail: pqi@parkinsons-qld.org.au

AUSTRALIA VICTORIA
Parkinson's Victoria, Inc.
20 Kingston Road, Cheltenham, Victoria 3192
(+61) 03 955 11122
Fax: (+61) 03 613 955 11310
Freecall: 1800 644 189 (Inside Australia)
E-mail: parksvic@satlink.com.au

WESTERN AUSTRALIA
Parkinson's Association of Western Australia (Inc.)
Centre for Neurological Support—The Niche
11 Aberdare Road, Suite B
Nedlands, WA 6009
(+61) 08 9346 7373
Fax: (+61) 08 9346 7374

AUSTRIA
Parkinson Selbsthilfe Österreich—
Dachverband
www.parkinson-sh.at, for more information contact:
sekretariat@parkinson-sh.at

CANADA
The Parkinson Society Canada
4211 Yonge Street, Suite 316
Toronto, Ontario, M2P 2A9
(+1) 416 227 9700
Fax: (+1) 416 227 9600
(800) 565-3000 (Inside Canada)
E-mail: general.info@parkinsons.ca
www.parkinson.ca
Has regional organizations to provide information, support services and specialized programs in their regions, including support groups you can join. For a list of the specific support and services available near you, visit the Web site.

HOLLAND
Parkinson Patienten Vereniging
Postbus 46, 3980 CA Bunnik, Netherlands
Tel: +31 30 656 1369, Fax: +31 30 657 1306
www.parkinson-verenigung.nl

ITALY
Associazione Italiana Parkinsoniani (AIP)
Via Zuretti, 35 – 20125, Milan
(+39) 02 6671 3111
Fax: (+39) 02 670 5283
www.parkinson.it

NEW ZEALAND
The Parkinsonism Society of New Zealand, Inc.
PO Box 10 392, Wellington
(+64) 04 472 2796
Fax: (+64) 04 472 2162
Freephone: 0800 473 4636 (Inside New Zealand)
E-mail: parkinsonsnz@xtra.co.nz

SOUTH AFRICA
Parkinson Association South Africa
Private Bag X36
Bryanston, 2021
(+27) 11 787 8792
Fax: (+27) 11 787 2407
E-mail: parkins@global.co.za

SPAIN
Parkinson Madrid
C/Andres Torrejon 18
Bajo 28014
Madrid
(+34) 91 434 0406
Fax: (+34) 91 434 0407
www.parkinsonmadrid.org
E-mail: parkinson@parkinsonmadrid.org

SWITZERLAND
Schweizerische Parkinsonvereinigung
Gewerbestrasse 12a, Postfach 123, CH-8132
Tel: +41 1 984 01 69, Fax: +41 1 984 03 93
www.parkinson.ch, for more information contact:
info@parkinson.ch

UKRAINE
HESED
For more information contact: *office@hesed.kiev.ua*

International Caregiver Information and Support Organizations

AUSTRALIA

Carers Australia
www.carersaustralia.com.au
(800) 242-636
Carers Australia represents the needs and interests of caregivers at the national level by

- *Advocating for carers' needs and interests in the public arena.*

- *Influencing government and stakeholder policies and programs at the national level through conducting research and pilot projects, giving presentations, and participating in a wide range of inquiries, reviews, and policy forums.*

- *Networking and forming strategic partnerships with other organizations to achieve positive outcomes for carers.*

- *Providing carers with information and education resources, undertaking community activities to raise awareness, and coordinating and facilitating joint work between the state and territory organizations on matters of national significance.*

CANADA

Canadian Caregiver Coalition
www.ccc-ccan.ca
The Canadian Caregivers Coalition helps identify and respond to the needs of caregivers in Canada. Links to organizations helpful to caregivers.

Caregiver Network, Inc.
(416) 323-1090
www.caregiver.on.ca
Based in Toronto, Canada, CNI's goal is to be a national single-information source to make your life as a caregiver easier.

UNITED KINGDOM

Carers UK
www.carersuk.org
The leading campaigning, policy, and information organization for carers; membership organization, led and set up by carers in 1965 to have a voice and to win the recognition and support that carers deserve.

UNITED STATES

. . . And Thou Shalt Honor
http://www.thoushalthonor.org/
The site for the acclaimed PBS caregiving documentary . . . And Thou Shalt Honor provides a variety of caregiving tools and resources.

Everyday Warriors
www.everydaywarriors.com
This site features numerous articles of interest to caregivers of all ages. Visit "Ask the Caregiver Coach," and "Caregivers Sound Off."

FamilyCare *America*, Inc.
1004 N. Thompson St., Suite 205
Richmond, VA 23230
(804) 342-2200
www.FamilyCareAmerica.com
FamilyCare America is dedicated to improving the lives of caregivers of the elderly, disabled, and chronically ill by creating a highly accessible resource where caregivers can:
- *better learn the process of caregiving*
- *receive help in managing their fears and concerns*
- *obtain resources for help with all aspects of caregiving*

Family Caregivers Alliance
690 Market Street, Suite 600
San Francisco, CA 94104
(800) 445-8106; 415-434-3388 FaxL (415) 434-3508
www.caregiver.org
E-mail: info@caregiver.org
Resource center for caregivers of people with chronic disabling conditions. The Web site provides information on services and programs in education, research, and advocacy.

National Alliance for Caregiving
4720 Montgomery Lane, 5th Floor
Bethesda, MD 20814
www.caregiving.org
The Alliance is a non-profit coalition of national organizations focusing on issues of family caregiving.

National Family Caregivers Association
10400 Connecticut Avenue, Suite 500
Kensington, MD 20895
(800) 896-3650
www.thefamilycaregiver.org
The Association supports, empowers, educates, and speaks up for the more than 50 million Americans who care for a chronically ill, aged, or disabled person.

National Quality Caregiving Coalition
750 First Street, NE
Washington, DC 20002-4242
(202) 336-5606
www.nqcc-rci.org
The NQCC is a coalition of national associations, groups, and individuals with interests in and active agendas that promote caregiving across all ages and disabilities throughout the lifespan.

Well Spouse Association
63 West Main Street—Suite H
Freehold, NJ 07728
(800) 838-0879
www.wellspouse.org
E-mail: info@wellspouse.org
A national, not-for-profit membership organization that gives support to wives, husbands, and partners of the chronically ill and/or disabled.

Insurance Issues

Geriatric Care Managers
National Association of Geriatric Care Managers
http://www.caremanager.org/

Medicare
http://www.medicare.gov/
General information about Medicare.

Medicare Rights Center
www.medicarerights.org
Having difficulties dealing with the health insurance maze? For those who have questions or problems regarding coverage, this not-for-profit, non-governmental website can provide some answers and suggestions.

End-of-Life Care

Aging with Dignity
www.agingwithdignity.org
A non-profit Web site that provides practical information, advice, and legal tools that can help you ensure that your wishes and those of your loved ones will be respected. Includes information about the Five Wishes document that helps you express how you want to be treated if you are seriously ill and unable to speak for yourself.

Last Acts Palliative Care Resource Center

http://lastacts.org/

Last Acts *is the largest campaign to improve care and caring near the end of life and is funded by The Robert Wood Johnson Foundation. This section of the Last Acts Web site focuses on practical information and tools on palliative care for both family members and health care professionals.*

Online Support Groups

CARE-Caregivers List

Because CARE is a closed list intended primarily for caregivers, please e-mail your request to join the list to owner Camilla Flintermann at flintec@muohio.edu.

It is helpful to tell briefly what your PD/caregiver situation is and to indicate where you live. You will be added, notified, and sent additional information when you are welcomed to this "virtual support group."

Parkinson's Information and Exchange Network Online (P-I-E-N-O)

http://www.parkinsons-information-exchange-network-online.com /parkmail/maillist.html

An international e-mail list and Web site about Parkinson disease.

Web Sites to Make Life Easier

The following Web sites offer extensive education and support services for caregivers.

CARE

www.geocities.com/pdcaregiver

Empowering Caregivers

www.care-givers.com

National Alliance for Caregiving
www.caregiving.org

National Family Caregivers Association
www.nfcacares.org

National Parkinson Foundation: Caregivers Forum
www.parkinsonscare.com

National Parkinson Foundation, Inc
www.parkinson.org

Parkinsonpoly
www.parkinsonpoly.com

The Parkinson's Disease Society
www.parkinsons.org.uk

Well Spouse Association
www.wellspouse.org

Glossary

A

Activities of daily living (ADL): personal hygiene, bathing, dressing, grooming, toileting, feeding, and transferring

Acute: state of illness that comes on suddenly and may be of short duration

Adult day care: centers that have a supervised environment where seniors can be with others

Advance directive: a legal document that states a person's health care preferences in writing while that person is competent and able to make such decisions

Ambulatory: able to walk with little or no assistance

Amnesia: complete or partial loss of memory

Analgesics: medications used to relieve pain

Antibiotics: a group of drugs used to combat infection

Anus: the opening of the rectum

Anxiety: a state of discomfort, dread, and foreboding with physical symptoms such as rapid breathing and heart rate, tension, jitteriness, and muscle aches

Apathy: a condition in which the person shows little or no emotion

Aphasia: a disorder that makes a person unable to speak, write, gesture, and/or understand written or spoken language (as in receptive aphasia)

Aromatherapy: use of essential oils of various plants to treat symptoms of diseases, improve sleep, and reduce stress by inducing relaxation

Artificial life-support systems: the use of respirators, tube feeding, intravenous (IV) feeding, and other means to replace natural and vital functions, such as breathing, eating, and drinking

Assessment: the process of analyzing a person's condition

Assisted living: housing for seniors offering independence, choice of services, and assistance with activities of daily living (ADLs), including meals and housekeeping

Atrophy: the wasting away of muscles or brain tissue

✑ B

Bedpan: a container into which a person urinates and defecates while in bed

Blepharospasm: involuntary clenching of the eyelids

Blood pressure: the pressure of the blood on the walls of the blood vessels and arteries

Body language: gestures that serve as a form of communication

Body mechanics: proper use and positioning of the body to do work and avoid strain and injury

Bradykinesia: literally, "slow movement"; one of the main symptoms of PD

✑ C

Calorie: the measure of the energy the body gets from various foods

Cataract: a condition (often found in the elderly) in which the lens of the eye become opaque

Catheter: a tube inserted into the bladder to collect or drain urine

Chronic: refers to a state or condition that lasts 6 months or longer

Colostomy: a temporary or permanent surgical procedure that creates an artificial opening through the abdominal wall into a part of the large bowel through which feces can leave the body

Congregate living: a type of independent living in which elderly people can live in their own apartments but have meals, laundry, transportation, and housekeeping services available

Conservator: a person given the power to take over and protect the interests of one who is incompetent

Constipation: infrequent or uncomfortable bowel movements

Contracture: shortening or tightening of the tissue around a joint so that the person loses the ability to move easily

D

Decubitus ulcer: pressure sore; bedsore

Defecate: to have a bowel movement

Defibrillator: a device that uses and electrical current to restore or regulate a stopped or disorganized heartbeat

Dehydration: loss of normal body fluid, sometimes caused by vomiting and severe diarrhea

Delusions: beliefs that are firmly held despite proof that they are false

Dementia: a progressive decline in mental functions

Depression: a psychiatric condition that can be moderate or severe and cause feelings of sadness and emptiness

Diffuse Lewy body disease: PD that has spread to include many parts of the brain and usually is characterized by both parkinsonism and dementia

Diuretics: drugs that help the body get rid of fluids

Dopamine: the primary chemical messenger of the basal ganglia; it is reduced in PD

Dopamine receptor: the part of the nerve cell in the striatum that receives dopamine

Draw sheet: a sheet folded widthwise to position under someone in bed to keep the linen clean and aid in transfers

Durable Power of Attorney: a legal document that authorizes another to act as one's agent and is "durable" because it remains in effect in case the person becomes disabled or mentally incompetent

Durable Power of Attorney for Health Care Decisions: a legal document that lets a person name someone else to make health care decisions after the person has become disabled or mentally incompetent and is unable to make those decisions

Dyskinesias: abnormal involuntary movements, usually associated with antiparkinson medication

Dysphagia: difficulty with or abnormal swallowing

Dystonia: in PD, tightness, spasm, or cramping of muscles; may also involve twisting or posturing of muscles

E

Edema: an abnormal swelling in legs, ankles, hands, or abdomen that occurs because the body is retaining fluids

End-of-dose failure: a loss of benefit from a dose of levadopa, typically at the end of a few hours

Estate planning: a process of planning for the present and future use of a person's assets

ꙥ F

Festination: tendency to propel forward as the patient accelerates with rapid, short steps

Foster care: a care arrangement in which a person lives in a private home with a primary caregiver and 4 or 5 other people

Freezing: inability to move or getting "stuck," as when the feet seem to be glued to the floor

ꙥ G

Gait: the manner in which a person walks

Geriatric: refers to care of older adults

Guardian: the one who is legally designated to have protective care of another person or of that person's property

ꙥ H

Hallucination: false perceptions (usually visual) of things that are not really there

Heimlich maneuver: a method for clearing the airway of a choking person

Hemiplegic: person who is paralyzed on one side of the body

Hospice: a program that allows a dying person to remain at home while receiving professionally supervised care

Hypomimia: the mask-like facial expression typical of PD

ꙥ I

Impaction: hardened stool mass blocking the bowel

Incontinence: involuntary discharge of urine or feces

Intravenous (IV): the delivery of fluids, medications, or nutrients into a vein

L

Laxative: a substance taken by mouth to produce a bowel movement in 6–8 hours

Levodopa: the chemical precursor of dopamine and the most effective treatment for PD

M

Mechanical lift: a machine used to lift a person from one place to another

Medic-Alert®: bracelet identification system. linked to a 24-hour service that provides full information in the case of an emergency

Medicaid: a U.S. health program that uses state and federal funds to pay certain medical and hospital expenses of those having low income, with benefits that vary from state to state

Medicare: the federal health insurance program in the U.S. for people 65 or older and for certain people under 65 who are disabled

Micrographia: the very small handwriting of someone with PD

Motor fluctuations: associated with the treatment of PD affecting ability to move; examples are wearing-off, on-off phenomenon, and dyskinesias

N

Neurotransmitter: a chemical messenger; dopamine is a neurotransmitter

Nutrition: a process of giving the body the key nutrients it needs for proper body function

O

Occupational therapy: therapy that focuses on the activities of daily living such as personal hygiene, bathing, dressing, grooming, toileting, and feeding

Off: the state of re-emergence of parkinsonian signs and symptoms when the medication's effect has waned

On: improvement in parkinsonian signs and symptoms when the medication is working at its peak

On–off phenomenon: unpredictable, usually abrupt changes in motor state

Oral hygiene: the process of keeping the mouth clean

Ostomy: surgery that creates an opening through the abdominal wall through which waste products can be passed

ᔣ P

Palilalia: stuttering or stammering speech in persons with PD

Paralysis: loss or impairment of voluntary movement of a group of muscles

Paranoia: a mental disorder characterized by delusions (often the belief that one is being persecuted)

Paraplegic: one who is paralyzed in (usually) the lower half of the body

Passive suicide: killing oneself through indirect action or inaction, such as no longer taking life-prolonging medications

Parkinsonian syndromes: disorders related to PD in that they are characterized by bradykinesia and sometimes rigidity, tremor, and balance problems, but have other chemical features and other pathology

Parkinsonism: the motor picture that makes up PD: bradykinesia, rigidity, tremor, balance, and gait problems

Pathogen: a disease-causing microorganism

Perineum: the area between the anus and the exterior genital organs

Physical therapy: therapy that focuses on gait, transfers, massage, and adaptive equipment

Pocketing: getting food caught between the cheek and the gum on the paralyzed side of face

Posey: a vest-like restraint used to keep a person from getting out of bed

Positioning: placing a person in a position that allows functional activity and minimizes the danger of faulty posture that could cause pressure sores, impaired breathing, and shrinking of muscles and tendons

Power of Attorney for Health Care: providing another person with the authority to make health care decisions

Pressure sore: a breakdown of the skin caused by prolonged pressure in one spot; a bed sore; decubitus ulcer

Prognosis: a forecast of what is likely to happen when an individual contracts a particular disease or condition

Prone: lying facedown

Prosthesis: an artificial body part, such as a tooth, an eye, a breast, leg, arm, hand, or foot

Q

Quadriplegia: paralysis of both the upper and lower parts of the body from the neck down

R

Range of motion (ROM): the extent of possible passive (movement by another person) movement in a joint

Rehabilitation: after a disabling injury or disease, restoration of a person's maximum physical, mental, vocational, social, and spiritual potential

Respite care: short-term care that allows a primary caregiver time off from his or her responsibilities

Retropulsion: tendency to fall backward

Rigidity: a tightness or increase in muscle tone at rest or throughout the entire range of motion of a limb, which may be felt as a stiffness by the patient

S

Sedatives: medications used to calm a person

Shock: a state of collapse resulting from reduced blood volume and/or blood pressure caused by burns, severe injury, pain, or an emotional blow

Sitz bath: a bath in which only the hips and buttocks are immersed into water or a medicated solution

Speech therapy: therapy that focuses on the treatment of disorders of speech, swallowing, and communication

Stroke: sudden loss of function of a part of the brain due to interference in its blood supply, usually by hemorrhage or blood clotting

Sundown syndrome: a period of severe confusion, agitation, irritability, and occasionally violence that can occur at the end of the day

Supine: lying on one's back

Support groups: groups of people who get together to share common experiences and help one another cope

Symptom: sign of a disease or disorder that helps in diagnosis

∿ T

Thalamotomy: surgical destruction of a small group of cells in the thalamus to abolish tremor on the side of the body opposite the surgery

Tracheotomy: surgical procedure to make an opening in a person's windpipe to aid in breathing

Tranquilizers: a class of drugs used to calm a person and control certain emotional disturbances

Transfer: movements from one position to another, for example, from bed to chair, wheelchair to car, etc.

Transfer belt: a device placed around the waist of a disabled person and used to secure the person while walking; gait belt

Transfer board (Sliding Board): polished wooden or plastic board used to slide a person when moving from one place to another, for example, bed to wheelchair or commode

Trapeze: a metal bar suspended over a bed to help a person raise up or move

Tremor: rhythmic shaking, usually of the hand (but also may affect the leg, lips, or jaw) that occurs at rest in PD; called postural or sustention tremor when extending the arms; action tremor when moving a limb

∿ U

Urinal: a container used by a bedridden male for urinating

Urinalysis: a laboratory test of urine

∿ V

Vaginal douche: a procedure to cleanse or medicate a woman's vagina by sending a stream of water into the vaginal opening

Vital signs: life signs such as blood pressure, breathing, and pulse

Void: to urinate; pass water

∿ W

Wearing-off: a loss of benefit from a dose of levodopa prior to time for the next dose

Index